Endorsements

In *Bod4God* Steve Reynolds launches a full-scale frontal assault in the ongoing American war with obesity. His weapons, solid biblical teaching and modern fitness principles, serve more effectively than any smart bomb or stealth warplane in the current battle against obesity. Reynolds' easy-to-understand, motivating plan can help even the most sedentary couch potato and is especially effective because it uses eternal wisdom from God's Word.

His plan helped to motivate our congregation of over 1,000 members to become healthier, leaner, and more joyful in just a short time and is now sweeping the globe. As a physician in a busy community practice, I have found it easy to share *Bod4God* with my patients as they fight their personal skirmishes with healthy living. Read *Bod4God* today, and enlist in the healthy army of the fit and faithful!

Darren Baroni, MD

Bod4God has produced more sustainable weight loss for its participants than any other program that I have been involved with in my twenty years as a dietitian. The focus on God and on losing weight for the right reasons was genuinely inspiring. The bonding, trust, and support of other participants helped keep the momentum going to achieve truly impressive results. Pastor Steve Reynolds is a great living example of God's power to transform.

Vivian Hutson, MA, MHA, RD, LD, FACHE (Lieutenant Colonel, U.S. Army)

Pastor Reynolds is a modern day prophet who strikes at the heart of the unhealthy lifestyle of most Americans and many members of the Christian community. His biblically based *Bod4God* is a credible program that could spark a movement toward weight control and healthier living. I heartily endorse this well-written, exciting book.

JAMES M. STERN, MD, FACS (Fellow of the American College of Surgeons)

Americans are in a fight for their health against a formidable "Goliath"—obesity. For years, the scientific community has told us what "stones" will weaken the giant—good nutrition and exercise. But translating bench-top research to everyday living is the challenge. What will powerfully propel those scientific stones? In *Bod4God*, Pastor Reynolds teaches us to be the "David." Armed with the slingshot of God's Word, you will launch healthy, up-to-date, scientific principles of exercise and nutrition to fight head-on the epidemic of obesity and topple the giant!

ELIZABETH P. BERBANO, MD, MPH (Fellow of the American College of Physicians; Certified, American Board of Internal Medicine)

It's been a blessing to partner with Pastor Reynolds and his congregation to provide Body & Soul as a key exercise strategy for the *Bod4God* program. In *Bod4God* there is a place for everyone to be successful. People of all ages and fitness levels have participated and seen improvements in cardiovascular fitness, strength, and flexibility. You will be encouraged and empowered by this book as you seek to improve your health and live a life of energy and vitality to God's glory.

JEANNIE BLOCHER, PRESIDENT, BODY & SOUL FITNESS MINISTRIES (Certified Faculty, American Council on Exercise; Group Fitness Specialist, Ken Cooper's Institute, Dallas, Texas)

I have seen patients turn life-threatening conditions into manageable ones or even experience full restoration through lifestyle change, including diet and exercise. Pastor Reynolds shows the powerful effects of faith and lifestyle change in his transformation from an obese man with illness requiring medication into a man unburdened by weight and illness.

ULRICH PRINZ, MD

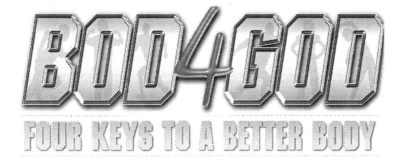

"*Bod4God* has produced more sustainable weight loss for its participants than any other program I have been involved with in my twenty
years as a dietitian."

--Vivian Hutson, MHA, RD, FACHE

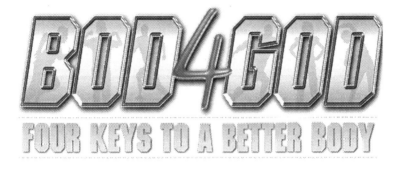

STEVE REYNOLDS

Fox News labeled Steve Reynolds "The Anti-Fat Pastor" after he lost
over one hundred pounds and launched a successful weight loss and
fitness program in his church with stunning results. In this book, he
reveals four keys to improve your health and lose weight.

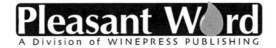

A Division of WINEPRESS PUBLISHING

Pleasant Word (a division of WinePress Publishing, PO Box 428, Enumclaw, WA 98022) functions only as book publisher. As such, the ultimate design, content, editorial accuracy, and views expressed or implied in this work are those of the author.

This book contains advice and information relating to health and medicine. It is not intended to replace medical advice and should be used to supplement rather than replace regular care by your physician. Readers are encouraged to consult their physicians with specific questions and concerns.

ISBN 13: 978-1-4141-1061-5
ISBN 10: 1-4141-1061-8
Library of Congress Catalog Card Number: 2007905080

Dedication

First, I dedicate this book to my God, who is the source of my life. I will spend the rest of my days on this earth honoring You with my body.

> *According to my earnest expectation and my hope, that in nothing*
> *I shall be ashamed, but that with all boldness, as always,*
> *so now also Christ shall be magnified in my body, whether it*
> *be by life, or by death.*
> (Phil. 1:20 KJV)

Second, I dedicate this book to Debbie, my wife, who is my partner in life. I will spend the rest of my days on this earth loving you with my body.

> *Who can find a virtuous woman? for her price is far above rubies.*
> *The heart of her husband doth safely trust in her, so that he shall*
> *have no need of spoil. She will do him good and not evil all the*
> *days of her life. Her husband is known in the gates, when he*
> *sitteth among the elders of the land.*
> (Prov. 31:10, 11-12, 23 KJV)

Third, I dedicate this book to Crystal, Sarah, and Jeremiah, my children, who are the inspiration for my life. I will spend the rest of my days influencing you with my body.

> *I have no greater joy than to hear that my children walk in truth.*
> (3 John 4 KJV)

Table of Contents

Acknowledgments

This was a TEAM project.

I greatly appreciate the group of people who helped me develop this book, including:

My parents, for always supporting me. I love you both very much.

My family, for sacrificing time without your husband and father while I worked on this book.

My wife, who helped me in various ways, I could not have done it without you!

My agent, Les Stobbe, my pastor, the late Jerry Falwell, my mentor, Elmer Towns, and my friend, Dave Earley, who helped me understand the media and publishing industry.

My assistant, Rindy Dowdy, who diligently helps me in so many ways.

My friends, Gary and Jana Moritz, who helped me shape the initial concepts for this project.

My writing assistant, Julie-Allyson Ieron with Joy Media, thank you for all you did to help this busy pastor and novice writer.

My proofreaders and researchers, Barbara Buis, Judy Byrd, Deni Carter, Sherry Chevalley, Brian Coss, Cary Eldred, Brenda Fahey, Grace Porter, Beth Ritter, and Kathie Scriven, who offered great suggestions and ideas.

My leaders and participants in the first ever Losing to Live Weight Loss Competition. You greatly motivated me.

My publisher for your guidance in producing a quality book.

My media contacts, thank you for helping to spread the *Bod-4God* message around the country and the world.

My readers, you honor me for taking time out of your busy lives to read this book.

THE

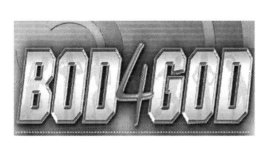

TRANSFORMATION

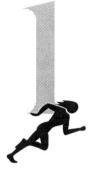

My Journey to...
a Bod4God

For by him were all things created, that are in heaven, and that
are in earth, visible and invisible, whether they be thrones, or
dominions, or principalities, or powers: all things were created by
him, and for him.
(Col. 1:16 KJV)

The headline on page one of *The Washington Post* on Monday, January 22, 2007, read, "Calling the Flock to God, Away from the Fridge: N.Va. Pastor Joins Ranks of Faithful Eyeing Scales." And the amazing thing was that the story was about me. Or rather about the weight loss journey I took, and the way I chose to share that journey with members of my congregation through a sermon series I titled *Bod4God*.

The media attention didn't stop with our regional newspaper, though. Almost immediately, the wire services picked up the story from the *Post*. Our local NBC affiliate sent a reporter and camera crew to cover my third *Bod4God* sermon and the kickoff of our church-wide weight loss challenge. And then I found myself being interviewed by the likes of Fox News Channel's Neil Cavuto; Christian Broadcasting Network; and even German, Canadian, and Swiss television.

The media attention had my mind reeling. This was my personal journey, and I'd wanted to share it with my congregation in the hopes that it would challenge a few of them to pursue a healthier lifestyle. But for the news of my weight loss program to go global, well, I was stunned—and frankly, a bit overwhelmed.

Weight was something I struggled with all my life. In first grade I weighed over a hundred pounds—104 to be exact. There were not many seriously overweight first graders in the world at that time. But I happened to be part of that club.

I'm told by my mother that when I was a baby, I had a sensitive stomach, and I would vomit a lot of my food. In fact, I didn't just vomit it, I projectile vomited. My mother obviously was successful at getting me to keep some of my food down. Somehow she overcame it; and if you know my mother, I'm sure she did it through lots of grease and sugar.

I grew up Southern, and proud of it. But I also grew up with that kind of diet and lifestyle, which included unhealthy eating patterns. So I weighed 104 pounds in first grade. I still have a report card that says, "Your son is thirty-six pounds overweight." I was one-third overweight. I wasn't a little bit overweight; I was a lot overweight.

One of the things I did to compensate for my weight was to get involved in sports, particularly football. I still have a picture of myself on the Sheffield Elementary School football field in my gold and black uniform.

I don't know how they do this today, but back in the day when I played, you played not only with the kids your age, but also your weight class. They didn't want these fat guys hurting these skinny guys, so they would look at you and ask, "How old are you?"

"I'm eight years old."

"How much do you weigh?" Your weight had to fall within a certain range for your age. If you weighed more than that range, they bumped you up to the next division where you would play with children older than you.

I never got to play with children my age. There were times I got bumped up two divisions, because I was so *healthy*. This ended up working to my advantage, because I became a pretty good football player. I was able to get half a dozen small colleges to recruit me to play football, and I ended up going to the greatest university in the world, Liberty University in Lynchburg, Virginia.

I was a four-year starter on Liberty's football team, and I was fortunate enough to go through college on a full football scholarship. I thank the Lord for that.

I also was fortunate enough to be able to use my football conditioning to my advantage. I worked out hard and was active. I would eat a lot, but I would exercise a lot, too; so at that stage of my life I got to a good playing weight and stayed in pretty good physical condition.

I Chose a Sedentary Lifestyle

I started playing football when I was seven or eight, and played all the way through until I was twenty-two. When I got done, here's what I said: "Nobody's ever going to make me run again in my life."

I've broken a lot of promises in my life. You probably have, too. Unfortunately, I kept that promise from age twenty-two to forty-eight. In all those years I never subjected myself to a regular exercise program.

I got out of college and went on to seminary. After seminary I was ordained. My beautiful bride Debbie and I were excited about the future together and our church-planting ministry calling. In fall 1982, Pastor Bob Eagy and I launched a new church just outside Washington, D.C.

In 2007 we celebrated our twenty-fifth anniversary of coming to Northern Virginia to plant a new church. Well, the good news is the church grew. The bad news is *I* also began to grow.

Part of the reason I began to grow was that I thoroughly love to work hard. But I also thoroughly love to come home after working hard and relax in my very own LaZBoy™ chair; I've had three over the course of my life, and I plan to go to the grave with some type of LaZBoy™ chair.

Some people on my ministry team want me to bring my chair to church and do a series on things I've taught in my home from my chair. Perhaps that would be a little over the top, but maybe not.

Anybody can sit in my chair when I'm not there, but when I come in, you're getting out of my chair and handing over the remote. It's that simple.

One of the things I could have taught from my chair was to eat ice cream every night. Yes, every night. I was addicted to ice cream. I'm not blame shifting, but I saw this pattern modeled throughout my childhood. To this day my dad eats ice cream every night. I've seen my dad eat a half gallon of ice cream at one time, but he doesn't look like I look because he does exercise regularly. So I would go home, see my wife, see the children, have a good time, sit in the chair—and eat ice cream.

There I was in my chair. The church was growing, and I was growing. In fact, I grew to 340 pounds. And I stayed there for years.

Impetus for Change

Then in 1999 I developed diabetes. I suppose that was part of the impetus it took to get me to look at my body and want to do something to change it. Diabetes is not always related to being overweight. Weight can be a contributor to it, but it also has a lot to do with heredity and your family history. My grandfather was a farmer; he was skinny and he was muscular (and to my knowledge, never overweight a day in his life). And yes, he was diabetic. My mother also is diabetic; but she is overweight. Then I discovered I had diabetes and I'm overweight. Although it's not always a weight issue, for me it was definitely related to weight.

God was working in my life, and God was telling me I needed to do something about this area in my life. Eventually, I began the journey of trying to improve my health. At first, this was an issue that was so personal it stayed between God and me. It was private. I was overweight, unhealthy, and painfully aware that I needed to make a permanent change in my life. I knew I couldn't do it without God's intervention, so I prayed and sought His direction. He is so gracious that He led me to a passage in His Word that directly addressed the issues I was facing. It gave me a step-by-step prescription for making this change in my life.

YOUR BODY IS MADE BY GOD AND FOR GOD

Once I began to follow it, I began to see results. Yes, I saw physical changes, but I also saw spiritual changes. My faith increased with each change I made and each pound I shed. It wasn't long before I knew it was my responsibility to share what I'd learned with my church and my community.

God began to work in my life, and I asked Him to give me something from His Word that would help me do what I needed to do when it came to health. It's His response to that request that I'll be sharing with you in the pages that follow. It's a message I've preached from my pulpit at Capital Baptist Church. It's a message I've had the opportunity to share with national and international audiences through news and talk shows. And I tell you, it works!

I Am a Loser

Today, I am proud to announce that I'm a loser; in fact, I want to see whole churches full of losers. My goal at Capital Baptist Church is to be the greatest losing church in America. I'd challenge you to be a loser, too.

I've lost over 100 pounds. I went from being diabetic to not being diabetic. Not every diabetic can get away from diabetes just by losing weight, but I was blessed that I was able to do that, and I am thankful for that. Now that I've lost the weight—it could change, but right now—I'm not battling diabetes.

I'm not about to judge anyone, least of all you, for I still need to lose more weight, and the difficult part will be keeping it off. It's never going to be easy; it's always going to be hard for me. This is a struggle in my life. But God has enlightened me to four keys in His Word that have helped get me to this point—and I intend to keep using them to help me stay on track in what I've come to call the *Bod4God* lifestyle.

Here's a chart that may help you get a handle on where your challenges are.

Your body is made by God and for God

CHART YOUR WEIGHT HISTORY

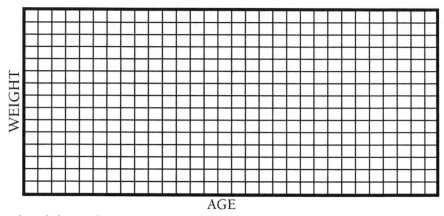

WEIGHT

AGE

What did you do to cause your weight to go up or down?

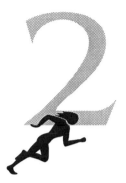

Losing to Live

Then Jesus said to His disciples, "If anyone desires to come after Me, let him deny himself, and take up his cross, and follow Me. For whoever desires to save his life will lose it, but whoever loses his life for My sake will find it."
(Matt. 16:24-25)

One of the things we're going to look at in this book is the fact that God created our bodies—hence the program name, *Bod4God*. The Bible says a lot about the body. In fact, the Bible uses the word *body* 179 times.

You may ask, "Is God really concerned about my body?" Well, He is concerned enough about your body that He would deal with it 179 times in the Bible. That is a lot of times for Him to deal with something in His Word. God didn't leave us without instruction. He didn't leave us without knowing how we can honor Him with our body. And so the Bible says we need to have a *Bod4God*. We need to take the body God has given us and use it for God. You see, your body, the Bible says, was created by God. My body was created by God.

Not only that, but the Bible tells us our bodies were created *for* God. God Almighty gave us life. And in giving us life, He not only created us, He created us for Himself.

Your life should be about Him. Your life should be about honoring Him. The Bible says, "For by him were all things created, that are in heaven, and that are in earth, visible and invisible, whether they be thrones, or dominions, or principalities, or powers: all things were created by him, and for him." (Col. 1:16 KJV)

More than a Weight-loss Plan

As I write, my purpose is to help you achieve a *Bod4God* lifestyle.

Now, although part of this book is going to be me describing how I lost over 100 pounds. This is going to be broader than weight loss. I want you to know that this is really going to be a study of what the Bible says about having a *Bod4God*—a body for and dedicated to God. For me, a big part of that has been dealing with my weight.

I realize that many of you don't need to lose weight. Whether you need to lose weight or not lose weight, this book is for you.

It's really about how you can have the keys here and now to have a better body. So I hope you will understand that as we go through this book.

Some of you who have bought this book have never met me. If you were to see me now you might expect to see a real skinny guy. But, I'm not skinny.

I don't want to be a skinny guy, okay. But I would like to be a skinnier guy. The point is that I am going to tell you out of my own life the steps I've taken in this journey of losing over 100 pounds. I want to tell you the keys I've used to take these steps in my life.

Again, this is not just coming out of some book on health, but this is literally my own story, the real steps I've taken in my life to help me lose the weight. So I hope this will be a help to you, as it was to me.

THE BOD 4 GOD
D.I.E.T. PLAN

Dedication: Honoring God With Your Body
Inspiration: Motivating Yourself For Change
Eat & Exercise: Managing Your Habits
Team: Building Your Circle Of Support

D-I-E-T Doesn't Stand for Diet

The next several chapters of this book are based on a series of messages I presented first in my own congregation. To help the audience remember the key points, I created an acrostic: DIET. I thought long and hard about this acrostic because there is a good reason I really didn't want to use it, because this teaching is not about a diet.

What I mean by that is a lot of times when we think about diet, we think about some crash diet or weight loss program we've heard about. This isn't about *diet* as much as it is about a change in *lifestyle*.

You see, I'm not on a short-term program, but I'm on a lifestyle program. I realize that only a small percentage of people keep off any weight they lose. It is wonderful to lose weight, but it is better to keep it off.

So I almost didn't use D-I-E-T because I didn't want to communicate to you that this is a short-term crash course. However, I decided to go ahead and do it because maybe it will help you remember the main points of this program.

D-I-E-T. The D stands for Dedication: honoring God with your body. The I stands for Inspiration: how do you motivate yourself to change? It's tough. The E stands for Eat and Exercise: habits that you have to build into your life. And then the T stands for Team: building your circle of support. You see, for me, I needed a team. I had to get my family on board with me. I had to get other people on board with me. I couldn't do it alone.

Later in the book, I'll describe the Losing to Live weight loss competition that grew out of this sermon series—and I'll make some suggestions about how you might begin a similar program in your church or community.

The theory here is that you are going to be much more successful in achieving a *Bod4God* lifestyle if you join up with other people and be part of a team for a significant period of time so you have a circle of support that can help you lose the weight. You need a team. It's a team effort. Most of us need help. Only a small percentage of us are disciplined enough to do this alone.

Self-denial

Anorexia has never been a problem in my life. It could have been me, but it's not me. Instead, I've struggled with weight gain—carrying more weight in my body than God ever intended for me to carry. This is something I have struggled with all my life.

As God began to stir in me about this issue in my life, I sensed I needed God to lead me through His Word. So I asked Him to show me in His Word something that would help me build a *Bod4God*. I prayed, "God, give me truth from Your Word that can help me to overcome this weight challenge in my life."

The passage God gave me was Matthew 16:24-25, "Then Jesus said to His disciples, 'If anyone desires to come after Me, let him deny himself, take up his cross, and follow me. For whoever desires to save his life will lose it, but whoever loses his life for My sake will find it.'"

My weight loss program, Losing To Live, comes, out of this passage in Matthew 16:24-25: "Then Jesus said to His disciples." To whom is Jesus talking? To His followers. So if you are a disciple, a learner of Jesus Christ, this statement is also being addressed to you: "If anyone desires to come after Me." Do you want to come after Him? The Bible says, "Let him deny himself."

You see, for me, the issue of living a healthy lifestyle was about me. I had to deal with self. I had to learn to deny myself. It required total dedication.

Dedication by Example

I had to say, okay, it's not about me. God didn't create this body for me; God created this body for Him. I've got to eat and I've got to exercise in a way that will bring honor and glory to Him, because it is His body, it is His temple.

When Jesus was in the Garden of Gethsemane, where He went to pray before He went to the cross, He prayed and asked the Father, "O My Father, if it is possible, let this cup pass from Me; nevertheless, not as I will, but as You will" (Matt. 26:39).

The answer was no, there is no other way for salvation. Only through Jesus and His death on the cross could we be saved.

Jesus, from a perspective of pain and suffering, didn't want to die on the cross, but He died to self, so to speak, to give His life to you and me. He prayed to the Father, "Your will be done, not Mine." It took dedication for Him to die on that cross for your sin and mine. But He did it because there was no other way.

Likewise, we have to deny ourselves. We have to take up His cross. I mean, what is the cross in your life? For me, part of that cross was food and exercise. I had to take up the cross, and I had to deny myself in an area that was difficult for me, if I wanted to follow Him.

So then, as much as we need to be willing to deny ourselves, even that much more we need to be willing to follow Jesus' example by taking up our crosses.

Live for Christ

After taking up our crosses, we have to be willing to follow Him. "Follow Me," Jesus says. The Bible says if we do it, we will find *true* life. It says, "Then Jesus said to His disciples, 'If anyone desires to come after Me, let him deny himself, and take up his cross, and follow Me. For whoever desires to save his life will lose it, but whoever loses his life for My sake will find it'" (Matt. 16:24-25).

Living your life for self is what it means to save your life. It means, "I'm going to live for self. I'm going to do what self wants to do." But you know what's going to happen? You're going to

lose your life. That means your life is not going to be a life of significance. And a life of significance not only makes a difference in
this world, but also in eternity. If you save your life and just live
for yourself, you'll lose your life.

But the Bible says—and this is what I had to do in my life—if
you will lose your life, "for My sake, you will find it." That means
saying, "Lord, I'm going to deny myself, I'm going to take up the
cross, and I'm going to follow You." That's losing your life. That's
saying, "I'm going to live for You."

Discover Real Life

Do you know what happens next? The Bible says if you deny
yourself you will discover true life. Do you really want to live? I'm
talking about *really* live? Then quit trying to live for self, and live
for Him. There you will find the abundant life Jesus talked about
in John 10:10, "The thief does not come except to steal, and to kill,
and to destroy. I have come that they may have life, and that they
may have it more abundantly."

God burned this into my heart. Matthew 16:24-25 is having
a huge influence on my life today, probably more than any other
passage.

What I learned that I didn't know, is that this passage is actually in the Bible six times. Jesus made this statement to multiple
people at multiple places. This was a major theme of His preaching. Everywhere He went, He wanted people to know, "Hey, you
want life?" Who doesn't want life? "Here's how you get it: Deny
yourself. Take up the cross and follow Me." So for me it was an
issue of being willing to lose to live.

THE

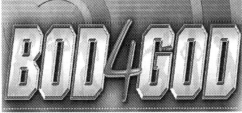

D-I-E-T
PLAN

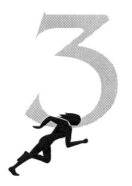

DEDICATION:
Honoring God
with Your Body

I say then: Walk in the Spirit, and you shall not fulfill
the lust of the flesh.
(Gal. 5:16)

I talk to a lot of people each week who call my office to talk about this program. Some weeks I'm on local and national—even international radio and TV. But one day a man who was at least an agnostic, perhaps even an atheist, asked me, "Don't you think it is possible to lose weight without God?"

I have to say it is. I mean, theoretically, a person can lose weight without God—people do it every day with secular programs. But for me, I could never lose weight without God. I needed God's help; I needed God's challenge and direction.

My journey began with dedicating myself to God. In Galatians 5:16, Paul called this concept walking in the Spirit. It means to allow the Holy Spirit to control you. The Bible says when you walk in the Spirit, you won't fulfill the lusts of the flesh. I had to learn to bring God's Holy Spirit into my life when it came to eating and exercise. I had to start depending on the Holy Spirit for guidance and especially for self-control in my eating habits.

The Bible says "the flesh is weak" (Matt. 26:41). That's the human aspect of who we are, our flesh. For me the flesh is particularly weak when it comes to eating and exercise. But the Bible says you won't fulfill the lust of your flesh if you will walk in the Spirit. That means you allow God, the Holy Spirit, to control you.

In other words, I had to learn to bring the Holy Spirit into my life when it came to what I ate and how I got my body moving. It was all part of acknowledging the indwelling of God's Holy Spirit in me.

I was one with the Holy Spirit when I preached, but I needed to add the Holy Spirit when I sat down to eat dinner. In fact, I might have needed the Holy Spirit more when I sat down to eat dinner than when I preached.

Here's the deal. We sometimes have a difference between belief and behavior, and we'll cover that issue in depth later. I had to bring those two together. For me, the first step was to dedicate this aspect of my life to God totally.

As part of that dedication to God, I had to learn to honor God with my body. We're going to talk about three things to do with your body. I'm going to walk through them step-by-step with you, and I'm going to show you how to honor God with your life. All three of these things come out of the book of Romans, which has a lot to say about the body.

**THE BOD 4 GOD
D.I.E.T. PLAN**

Dedication: Honoring God With Your Body

I

E

T

Number One: Dedicate Your Body

Dedicate your body! You've got to come to God and say, "God, I want to dedicate my body to You." Romans 12:1-2 says, "I beseech you therefore, brethren, by the mercies of God, that you present your bodies a living sacrifice, holy, acceptable to God, which is your reasonable service. And do not be conformed to this world, but be transformed by the renewing of your mind, that you may prove what is that good and acceptable and perfect will of God."

You see, the Bible says here, "I am begging you earnestly," that's what *beseech* means. Paul is pleading with us. He is saying, "I am begging you earnestly to do this." What does God want us to do? Present our bodies. We need to come today and we need to present our bodies to God.

How do we do that? Number one, the Bible tells us to do that as living sacrifices. We say, "God, I want to give my life to You; I want to sacrifice my body for You. I want to be a living sacrifice."

Second, it says "holy." That's right. God says, "I want you to present your body to Me as holy." It goes on to say it's not only a living sacrifice, not only holy, but also doing what is acceptable to God. Our prayer needs to be, "God, I want to do with my body only what fits into the standard of what is acceptable to You." Remember, this is only our "reasonable service." God gave it all for us, so why shouldn't we give our all for Him?

The Bible tells us not to be conformed to this world. When it comes to losing weight, this is a big issue. What's the world like? In the world today, a large percentage of the people are unhealthily overweight.

But the Bible says be not conformed to the world, but be transformed, be changed, by the renewing of what? Your mind. You have to have a different mindset, and that mindset is to know what is good and acceptable and perfect when it comes to the will of God.

So, number one, dedicate your body. Your body is not for the gratification of self, but rather for the glorification of God. Our bodies were not given to us so we could do what we want to do with them.

We hear people say, "It's my body; I can do what I want to with it." No, it's not your body. And, no, you can't do what you want with it.

We hear this message particularly in the abortion debate. While that's outside the scope of this particular message, the principle is the same.

God gave us bodies to honor Him—they're not our own to do with as we please. Unfortunately, I've preached sermons on that and dealt with that, the whole time being as fat as could be.

Philippians 3:19 talks about people "whose god is their belly." Our belly is all about self and doing what self wants to do. This is why for me it started out with denying myself. I had to be willing to deny myself, because my god was my belly.

Again, the disconnect between belief and behavior. If you had asked me, "Hey, what's your body for?" I would have responded, "Oh, it's for God." That was what I believed, but my behavior didn't reflect that in my lifestyle. You know, if you really believe something, you're going to do it, if you really believe it. But although I said it, I didn't do it, so the truth is I didn't really believe it. You've got to bring belief and behavior together. And for me, that was a big struggle.

I had to realize my body was not for the gratification of self, but my body was for the glorification of God. Your body is about God. It was created by God and for God, and like Paul says in Philippians 1:20, he wanted Christ to be magnified in his body.

I wanted to bring belief and behavior together, and what was needed was dedication.

Number Two: Discipline your Body

Romans 6:11 tells us, "Likewise you also, reckon yourselves to be dead indeed to sin, but alive to God in Christ Jesus our Lord." There's that concept again of losing yourself, dying to self, being dead to sin, but alive to God. The whole concept there is one of dying to self, dying to sin, and denying self, and being alive unto God through Jesus Christ.

> *Therefore do not let sin reign in your mortal body, that you should obey it in its lusts. And do not present your members as instruments of unrighteousness to sin, but present yourselves to God as being alive from the dead, and your members as instruments of righteousness to God.*
>
> —Rom. 6:12-13

YOUR BODY IS MADE BY GOD AND FOR GOD

What does "members" refer to? It is about body parts. Do not yield your body parts unto sin, "But rather, yield yourself unto God, as though alive from the dead, and your members," your body parts, "as instruments of righteousness unto God."

You see, I had to come to the point where I had to discipline my body parts. I want to invite you to join me in dedicating your body parts to God. The Bible says don't yield your members, your body parts, to sin, but yield your body parts to God.

What are some specific body parts? Let's start at the feet and work up, how about that?

Your Feet
The Bible says your feet need to be dedicated to God. Romans 10:15 says, "How beautiful are the feet of those who preach the gospel of peace, Who bring glad tidings of good things." What are you supposed to do with your feet? The Bible says if you want beautiful feet, beautiful feet are those feet that preach the gospel.

You need to dedicate your feet to God, and say, "God, with my feet, wherever I go, I want to be a witness for You, whether I go to church, to my job, to the grocery store, or anywhere else. God, as I'm walking, these feet that You've given me are going to be feet that I'm going to use to be a witness for You. I'm not going to take these feet to places where I can't honor You. I'm not going to allow these feet to go to places that would displease You. I dedicate my feet to You, and wherever I go with these feet, I am going to be a witness for You, because I want to have beautiful feet."

Would you right now present your feet to God? Give them to the Lord; let Him have them.

"Here they are, God. Right here, Lord."

Your Sexuality
Now on to another part of your physical body. We are sexual beings; God has given us sexual organs. But disciplining ourselves as instruments of righteousness to God also means disciplining our sexuality. It's important to realize your mind is your most influential sexual organ. If you want to have proper control of your

other sexual organs, you need to discipline your mind with pure thoughts.

The Bible says, "For this is the will of God, your sanctification: that you should abstain from sexual immorality; that each of you should know how to possess his own vessel in sanctification and honor" (1 Thess. 4:3-4). You see, all sex outside of marriage is sin. I'd encourage you to say out loud right where you are just now, "God, I'm not going to sin with my sexuality. I'm not going to get involved in fornication. I'm not going to get involved in adultery. God, I right now present my sexuality to You. God, You made sex; You're pro-sex."

One of the coolest things about God is He created sex. He is a cool God, but He gave some guidelines. He says sexual activity should only occur between a husband and a wife. He said you can have sex, but you've got to find a husband, or find a wife, and be faithful to your husband, or be faithful to your wife.

"God, I present my sexuality to You."

Your Emotions
The next area I feel is especially important to discipline, especially if you are overweight, is emotion.

A particular area in need of discipline here is bitterness. One of the greatest damages that we do to our bodies is bitterness. Your body was not designed to house bitterness. Bitterness is like a poison. It will destroy your body.

As Hebrews 12:15 says, "Looking carefully lest anyone fall short of the grace of God; lest any root of bitterness springing up cause trouble, and by this many become defiled."

Medical science corroborates that biblical truth, suggesting that bitterness is a contributing factor to many diseases.

Some of you are eating right, you're exercising right, and you may still die young because you are a bitter person. Bitterness will kill you. You may die early unless you learn a lifestyle of forgiveness. Remember, forgiveness is not an option, but a command, as Paul explained in Ephesians 4:32, "And be kind to one another, tenderhearted, forgiving one another, even as God in Christ forgave you."

"God, I want to present my emotions to You. I want to learn a lifestyle of forgiveness."

A BOD4GOD CLOSE-UP:

Terry and Paula Menteer

Paula was driving down the interstate between Virginia and Pennsylvania (where she was going to help her nursing home-bound mother) when her favorite radio station FM 105 WAVA played an ad for the Losing to Live weight-loss competition. She recalls, "I had come to a point where I felt I was out of control with my eating. When I heard about it on 105, I began praying about it. I told the Lord that if I heard this on my way home, I would look into it." Sure enough, the ad played again during Paula's return trip. So she looked it up on the Internet and talked with her husband Terry (a retired Marine) about joining.

The couple drives forty miles each Sunday evening to attend the sessions—which is only part of the way they're demonstrating their dedication. Terry explains, "When we came into it, it was not to lose a little bit of weight and then go back to what we were doing before. We came into it as a life-changing experience—forever, not just for a few months."

They describe their new eating plan as all about "portion control—eating healthy and eating less." Paula is excited that these new choices have allowed her to discontinue her blood pressure pills, at her doctor's direction.

In twenty weeks Paula lost eighteen pounds and Terry lost thirty-one.

Your Hands

The next body part for discussion is your hands. The Bible says, "Cleanse your hands, you sinners" (James 4:8). What do you do with your hands? I mean, for me, part of my sin was picking up the wrong kind of food and eating it.

Maybe it's you taking your hands and picking up a cigarette, or marijuana, or something like that. Maybe it's touching somebody who is not your spouse with your hands. "Cleanse your hands, you sinners." Dedicate your hands to God.

"God, I'm going to honor You with my hands. I'm going to please You with my hands."

Your Mouth

The next object of personal discipline is your mouth. Here I'm not even talking about what you put in your mouth, but instead what comes out of your mouth. Proverbs is full of exhortations to discipline your speech. James 3:10 says, "Out of the same mouth proceed blessing and cursing. My brethren, these things ought not to be so." Of course, discipline isn't complete with only what comes out of your mouth. We also must discipline what goes into our mouths.

Proverbs 23:2 says, "Put a knife to your throat if you are a man given to appetite." Wow! You may ask, "Does God really want me to cut my throat?" No, of course not. But what He's trying to tell you is: hey, overeating is serious, because it destroys your health. *When you love potlucks more than God, it's serious.* When "all you can eat" is the way you live your life, it's serious.

What the Bible is saying is that if you are prone to gluttony, you need to take drastic measures to bring your appetite under control. If necessary, take drastic measures to get your appetite under control. I'm a man given to appetite. Therefore, I've got to take drastic steps to control what goes into my mouth.

Discipline your mouth. Will you give your mouth to God?

"Lord, You reign right here. Here's my mouth, I'm giving it to You."

Your Eyes

Next we will discuss the importance of disciplining your eyes. David said, "I will set no wicked things before my eyes" (Ps. 101:3). What about that pornography? "God, I want to give You my eyes.

I want to present them right now to You. Here are my eyes, God. I dedicate them to You. I will set no wicked thing before my eyes."

Ladies, I know clothes are important, I understand all that, but I just want you to know something about men, because you may not realize this. Men and women are not the same. We men are turned on visually. You ladies, most of you can't relate, because you're different. You have to be touched. That's how God made you. That's why 1 Timothy 2:9 says, "Women, adorn yourselves in modest apparel." Again, modest apparel.

You may say, "Well, you men need to get yourselves under control." You're right, we need to get ourselves under control. But please help us with what you wear. Adorn yourself in modest apparel.

And then, take it off for your husband. That's fine. But otherwise, dress modestly. Help us out a little bit. Pray for us.

"God help me keep my eyes pure, and show me if I'm causing others to stumble in this area."

Your Ears

Let's move on to the need to discipline your ears. Give God your ears. God says, listen to Him with your ears. Incline your ears to God. And listen to people. God says, "Be swift to hear, slow to speak" (James 1:19). Consider the fact that God gave you two ears and one mouth; maybe He wants you to listen twice as much as you talk.

We all need somebody to listen to us at times. That's a ministry you can have with people, with your ears.

"God, I'll be a listener."

Your Mind

The next body part is another really big one: your mind. The Bible says, "Let this mind be in you which was also in Christ Jesus" (Phil. 2:5). Our goal should be to always have the mind of Christ, to ask, "What would Jesus do?"

The standard for our thought lives is Philippians 4:8: "Whatever things are true, whatever things are noble, whatever things are just, whatever things are pure, whatever things are lovely, whatever things are of good report, if there is any virtue and if there is anything praiseworthy—meditate on these things."

"God, take my mind and set it on things that bring you glory."

Your Heart

Lastly, discipline your heart. Romans 10:9 says, "If you confess with your mouth the Lord Jesus and believe in your heart that God has raised Him from the dead, you will be saved." Dedication to God begins by being a follower of Christ, by forming a relationship with Christ. The way you form that relationship with Christ is to realize you are a sinner; you have broken God's laws. We have all broken the Ten Commandments. You have lied; you have stolen; you have dishonored your father and your mother; you have put other things ahead of God; you have misused the name of God.

We have all broken God's laws. The Bible says because of that we all deserve hell. Then Jesus came, and Jesus died on the cross for our sins. He was buried, and on the third day He rose from the grave to give us eternal life. The Bible says to be saved you have to confess it with your mouth, and believe it in your heart. That's where dedicating yourself to God begins.

Then make sure your heart and your lips are together. Jesus talked about people who honor Him with their lips, but their heart is far from Him. Dedicate your heart to God.

If you would like to receive Christ as your personal Lord and Savior, tell God in the following prayer:

"Dear God, I am a sinner. Because of my sin, I deserve to spend eternity in hell. I believe Jesus died on the cross, was buried, and rose from the grave for my sins. I therefore turn from my sins and put my faith in Jesus Christ to get me to heaven. Thank You for saving me today, and help me to serve You the rest of my life. In Jesus' name, Amen."

Deliver Your Body

One day you're going to stand before God and you'll be required to give an account of your life. Romans 14:10-12 says, "But why do you judge your brother? Or why do you show contempt for your brother? For we shall all stand before the judgment seat of Christ. For it is written: 'As I live, says the LORD, Every knee shall bow to Me, And every tongue shall confess to God.' So then each of us shall give account of himself to God." The big things for which you're going to give an account of include:

- You're going to give an account of your *time.* We all have the same amount of time, and we're going to have to answer God for how we have used our time.
- You're going to have to give an account of your *talents.* What did you do with the talents that God gave you?
- You're going to have to give an account of your *treasure.* You're going to have to answer God about your money and what you did with your money.
- You're going to have to give account for your *temple,* what you did with your body. One day you are going to deliver your body to God, and say, "God, here I am, standing in judgment before You." And God's going to put that light on your time, and your talent, and your treasure, but He's also going to look at your temple.

2 Cor. 5:10 says, "For we must all appear before the judgment seat of Christ, that each one may receive the things done in the body, according to what he has done, whether good or bad."

Looking Ahead

In the next chapter, we're going to look a lot more at what it means to say our bodies are the temple of God. We'll examine the next key that will motivate you to work toward having a *Bod4God.*

To be sufficiently motivated, we need to know our bodies are God's temples. So dedicate yourself, discipline yourself, and make good plans now to deliver yourself to God—wholly and completely.

Then you'll be ready for the next step. But for now, let's pray together as we dedicate ourselves to honoring God with our bodies.

> *"Father, I love You, and I thank You for Your Word. You are an awesome Creator. I dedicate my entire body to You. Please help me to completely honor You with my time, talents, treasure, and temple. In Jesus' name, Amen."*

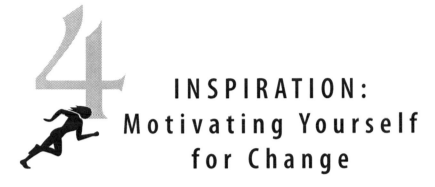

INSPIRATION:
Motivating Yourself
for Change

The thief does not come except to steal, and to kill, and to destroy.
I have come that they may have life, and that they may have it
more abundantly.
(John 10:10)

A lot of us know we should get healthier, but the problem is we're not motivated to do it. In this section we'll discuss how to get inspired and how to stay motivated for a healthy lifestyle. In this chapter we'll talk about key number two for getting a better body: Inspiration: Motivating Yourself For Change.

As we begin, let me remind you that your body was created by God and for God. This is the foundation of *Bod4God*. Your body was created by God—God made you for Himself. The Bible says, "For by him were all things created, that are in heaven, and that are in earth, visible and invisible, whether they be thrones, or dominions, or principalities, or powers: all things were created by him, and for him" (Col. 1:16, KJV). Key phrases here are *by Him* and *for Him*.

You see, you were created by Him. God gave you life. And God today sustains your life. God is the one allowing your heart to beat right this moment. God is the one allowing your lungs to function today. God is allowing your brain to function. God has given you life. God made you, and God is sustaining you in life.

The Bible tells us God made us, not for us, but for Him. You were made *for Him.* Your life and my life are to be about honoring Him. We're to have a *Bod4God.*

THE BOD 4 GOD
D.I.E.T. PLAN

Dedication: Honoring God With Your Body
Inspiration: Motivating Yourself For Change
E
T

Why Does God Care About Our Bodies?

You might be wondering, *What's a church, or what's a pastor, doing talking about physical things?* I think this is why the world gets intrigued by what I've discovered about having a *Bod4God*—and why the media has been so interested in what I preached and continue to teach about it. But the truth is what we're talking about is not just physical, it's something spiritual.

The Bible uses the word *body* 179 times. It's as if God is telling us, "Now listen, I'm the One who made you, I made you for Me." And He didn't leave us on the earth without direction. He told us in His Word what He expects from us when it comes to the body. And this concept is all about the body God has given to us. The purpose of this book is to help you achieve a *Bod4God* lifestyle. I know many of you don't need to lose weight. Yet, the truth is everybody needs to hear this message, because what I'm writing about is going to help you in every area of your life. These are transferable concepts.

I want to tell you what inspired me to lose weight. These chapters aren't coming out of some other source or curriculum, or whatever. I'm telling you how I have used what I'm teaching to lose over 100 pounds. You can take these keys and apply them to whatever other areas God is dealing with in your life.

For example, in this chapter we're going to talk about inspiration: how to inspire yourself, how to motivate yourself to change.

Your body is made by God and for God

Maybe you don't need to change in the area of weight. Maybe you are doing just fine in that area, but you're trying to do something better in another area of life. Most people have goals concerning areas they'd like to improve on. No doubt you're trying to improve *something*.

You can take almost everything I've discovered and apply it to whatever area you want to see yourself improve on. That's what I mean by transferable concepts—they can be applied to another situation, no matter what you're dealing with. I also want to emphasize this is about being healthy, not necessarily about losing weight, and all of us want to be healthy. I ask you to keep that in mind as you read on.

A Continuing Healthy Lifestyle

Remember, the four keys to a better body fit into the acrostic D-I-E-T. The first was Dedication. Now, we turn our attention to key two: Inspiration. It's the second letter in our acrostic, DIET.

Remember that in this book we're not talking about a diet in the sense of a short-term fix. We're talking about a healthy lifestyle that continues after any weight loss you may achieve. When most of us think of the word *diet* we think of something negative, because who wants to be on a diet?

We also think of something short-term, "I'm going to diet and lose ten pounds." So when you think about it, think about D, that is Dedication, I, which is Inspiration, E, which is Eat and Exercise, T, which is Team. The reason we're going to use this acrostic is because it might help you to remember it.

God's Word has Something to Say

I believe God gave Matthew 16 to me when I needed it, because although I had seen this passage before, I never thought about it in the context God showed it to me recently. Matthew 16:24-25 quotes Jesus as saying, "If anyone desires to come after Me, let him deny himself, and take up his cross, and follow Me. For whoever

A Bod4God Close-up:
Karen and Laura Cunningham

This mother/daughter team is finding in each other inspiration and encouragement in the weight-loss journey. Karen is a single mom employed as a nanny; her daughter Laura is fifteen. After hearing about Bod4God on Christian radio, they now attend Capital Baptist Church's 8:15 A.M. service before going to their own church's 10 A.M. service. Laura says, "I've made small, simple changes, which is awesome! The fact it's just Mom and me at home, our whole household has changed. It is easier not having temptations in the house." She is excited about the changes in her mom: "Mom was always very tired. She started exercising, and she's now healthier and happier."

Karen describes her motivation as deeper than body image or physical health. "To think I have been a Christian for thirty years and I had never connected watching the kinds of food I eat—the big steaks, considering quick trips to McDonalds a 'hot meal,'—with being God's temple. What I was doing to myself was showing a bad example to my daughter and dishonoring God."

The pair now swims together and works out regularly. Once they reach their weight-loss goals, they'll celebrate: "Our reward and celebration is not about food—we won't celebrate with chocolate cake!"

In twenty weeks Laura lost twenty-four pounds and Karen lost thirty-six.

desires to save his life will lose it, but whoever loses his life for My sake will find it."

Now, in chapter three we looked at the first part of that verse as we focused on dedication: honoring God with your body. Now we're going to turn to the second part of that verse, which is about having life. Jesus said that if you save your life, you will lose it.

If you live your life for yourself, saying, "I'm going to live the way I want to live, do what I want to do," you will lose your life, meaning your life will amount to nothing of eternal significance. If you want to live a life of significance and not just simply strive for some worldly success, if you want to leave a legacy that means something, you need to lose your life. In other words, give up your life to Him. Honor Him with it. Jesus said if you save your life you will lose it. But if you will lose your life—and here are the key words, *"For My sake"*—you will find life.

Jesus stated that the Christian life means losing to live. Again, this statement is repeated six times in the Bible. Remember, this was a theme of His preaching. And this is the passage God gave to me to focus more of my time and energy toward losing weight and getting healthier.

I suppose this spoke to me so powerfully because when it came to inspiration for me, it was all about life. I wanted to experience the fullness Jesus promises in John 10:10 where He says, "The thief does not come except to steal, and to kill, and to destroy. I have come that they may have life, and that they may have it more abundantly."

The thief is Satan. You know what Satan wants to do in your life? He has an agenda for your life, and it includes this: he wants to steal from you, he wants to kill you, and he wants to destroy you.

I realized the thief was coming into my life through food and lack of exercise, and he was stealing from me. He was killing me. I was diabetic, and this disease will destroy your health. He was seeking to destroy me. *The way Satan was killing me was with a knife and a fork.* He was doing a really good job at pursuing his goals for me, because diabetes kills.

But I wanted to live. I wanted to live here and now receiving the promise Jesus gave, "I am come that they might have life and that they might have it more abundantly."

What I wanted was a better quality of life and a better quantity of life. I wanted to lose myself so I could live. You have to find out what is going to inspire you, but this is the foundation of what inspired me to get on this pathway of getting healthy, and it is what keeps me on this pathway. I want to live. I want to live a better life, and I want to live a longer life down here on earth. Of course, I look forward to heaven. I just don't want to rush it.

Eternity is a long time, and I'm looking forward to being there forever, but I want to experience life with my wife and family on this earth as long as I can.

An Example from Fatherly Love

I don't know if any father could love his children more than I love my three children. I'm sure we could debate about that, dads. But I promise you, I don't know how anybody could love their kids more than I love my kids. Crystal, Sarah, and Jeremiah are all precious to me.

I don't know what might happen with Capital Baptist Church in the coming years—what my legacy will be in that institution—but I'm telling you I measure my success in my life by how my children serve God. They are my first ministry. That's just how it is. I love my wife and three children more than anything in this world.

Today my children are young adults. Yet, even young adults and middle-aged adults look to their parents for guidance in life. You might want to keep that in mind if your children are grown.

I want to be on this earth as long as I can be to influence them. I'm not one of these guys who says, "You're eighteen. You're on your own." No, they're never going to get rid of me. We're beyond the control phase, but I'm going to influence those children until my dying breath, to the best of my ability.

I want to see my grandchildren. I want to influence them. I even want to see my great-grandchildren. I want to know them. I'm probably asking too much for great-great-grandchildren. But, I'm just saying, I want to live.

Somebody might be saying, "You're having a midlife crisis." I'm not having a midlife crisis; *I'm having a midlife revival.* If you're reaching mid-life, I'd suggest the same revival for you. Your most fruitful and productive years can be ahead of you. Don't waste them.

As I write, I'm preparing to celebrate twenty-five years of coming to the Washington, D.C., area. I'm getting ready for the next twenty-five. I want to live. That's what inspires me. What inspires you?

Think about it. How can you motivate yourself for change? God used the concept of "Quit digging your grave with a knife and fork," and it comes from a book written by a person who's on my team. Again, part of doing this is not doing it alone. One of the men on my team doesn't even know me, and I don't know if I'll ever meet him. But he has made an impact on my life. His name is Mike Huckabee and at the time I wrote this book, he was the governor of Arkansas. He lost over 100 pounds and wrote a book called *Quit Digging Your Grave With a Knife and Fork*.

Some of us go get books that we don't read. I do that sometimes, and perhaps you do too. But here's a book, if you never read it, just look at the cover every once in a while. The book is great—I've read every word of it three times. But the cover is the greatest—because that title will remind you of what you're doing to yourself. This book was a major catalyst that helped me seriously start on a path to losing weight.

God used this man to make a difference in my life. After reading his book, I lost a lot of weight and went from being diabetic to not being diabetic. It reminded me that I want to live.

How Do You Motivate Yourself to Change?

I had to find the motivation for change. How was I going to inspire myself? I chose to focus on my desire to live. Perhaps the best thing about life being your motivation is it's a permanent sort of goal. It wasn't just pounds I wanted to lose—I wanted to live a longer life and a better life on this earth. And my chances of living longer increase when I'm healthy. I know I can have a better quality of life if I am healthier. Life inspires me more than anything else.

Whether you are married or single, you may have children or other loved ones who can serve as part of your motivation for change. Or God may use another motivator for you. Prayerfully ask Him for His help.

I want to emphasize again that this is not simply about losing weight. This is about changing your life. What area do you need to change? I promise you, these four keys I'm going to share apply to any area of change. So maybe it's not losing weight for you. Maybe it's something else. You take every one of these points and plug them into your problem, and I guarantee you it will help you. But this is my journey. This is what I've done and what I am doing in this area of change.

Rely on God

The number one way for me to stay motivated is to rely on God. You see, for me, I need God to help me. Earlier I shared with you that we've had a lot of people contact me about this information and about our weight loss competition. I've tried to talk to as many of them as possible.

I made it a priority because I was trying to learn what was going on in the lives of others who were also trying to lose weight. I was trying to connect with the culture and see what fellow weight-loss participants were dealing with, so I could make this message practical and relevant to readers.

As I told the agnostic caller, "There are lots of people who have lost weight and didn't have God to help them. But for me, I needed God." I couldn't do this by myself. I needed someone, God, who is greater than I am, to help me. I needed to experience Philippians 4:13 where Paul said, "I can do all things through Christ who strengthens me." I can do all things, and to me that meant I can get healthy through Christ who strengthens me.

What do you need to put in that spot among the "all things" Christ can strengthen you to accomplish? Is it cigarettes? Is it poor management of your time or other resources? Is it dealing with bitterness and anger? There are so many areas where you can apply this.

YOUR BODY IS MADE BY GOD AND FOR GOD

What would you put there? For me it was, "I can get healthy through Christ who strengthens me." I needed Christ to strengthen me. I knew I was weak in my flesh. In Matthew 26:41 Jesus says, "Watch and pray, lest you enter into temptation. The spirit indeed is willing, but the flesh is weak."

Many times throughout my life I had said, "I've got to get healthy. I've got to lose weight. I've got to exercise." My spirit has always wanted to do that, but my flesh was weak. I had to learn to pray specifically for the power of the Holy Spirit to fill my life in the area of health.

The Bible says, "Walk in the Spirit, and you shall not fulfill the lust of the flesh" (Gal. 5:16). God had a solution for the weak flesh I had, and still have—to walk in the Spirit, more specifically, to walk in the Spirit at the dinner table. I made a conscious decision to "walk in the Spirit at the dinner table."

I had to take the filling of the Holy Spirit that I experienced at church and in other spiritual activities to the table where I ate. I had to know He was there with me, giving me strength, whenever and wherever I ate.

Like the Holy Spirit had to be part of my meals, the Holy Spirit also had to be part of me getting moving in exercising. It was about the Holy Spirit controlling me in those areas and being filled with the Holy Spirit.

Refine Your Attitude

Number two, you've got to refine your attitude. I had to deal with my attitude. The Bible says, "As he thinks in his heart, so is he" (Prov. 23:7). Your attitude, not your aptitude, determines your altitude in life.

I knew what I needed to do. I had the aptitude to do this; I didn't possess the attitude to do it. My weight issues were destroying me. All of us have some unhealthy attitudes to work through.

Unhealthy Attitudes Toward Your Body
Do you reject your body? Some of us look at our bodies and say, "God, You messed up when you made me." Have you ever felt like that? Self-esteem is a big problem for most overweight people.

Some of that may come from good old Barbie, ladies. My girls never had a Barbie. I wouldn't dare buy one of my kids a Barbie. I didn't want my young ladies to be picking up some 36-24-36, no acne image they would carry with them through their childhood and beyond. Parents, keep them out of your house. Same for Ken. I didn't look like Ken growing up. Did you guys? Okay, I wasn't a Ken. And I wasn't G.I. Joe either. I was more like Mr. Potato Head; that's about what I looked like growing up, Mr. Potato Head.

Many of us don't necessarily like our bodies. Knowing that, some of us have the unhealthy attitude that we can perfect what we have. Some of us go too far in this. We feel somehow—through whatever means available—we can buy ourselves the *perfect* body. We have surgeries to make us look different. We exercise to excess. We watch every morsel that goes into our mouths. Our aim is to gain for ourselves the perfect body.

I want to be honest with you: I'm not trying to get perfect, but I am trying to get a healthy body. We can begin to idolize our bodies if we put too much priority on them. This is an unhealthy, ungodly attitude that we need to change.

But there's another unhealthy attitude: you can neglect your body. This is what most people do. Most of us have neglected our bodies; we haven't made caring for our bodies a big enough priority.

A Healthy Respect for the Body God Created
For me, the healthy attitude was that I wanted to maximize my body. It wasn't about rejecting it; it wasn't about perfecting it; it wasn't about neglecting it. I just wanted to, and still want to, maximize my body. Psalm 139:14 says, "I am fearfully and wonderfully made." This body God gave to me is incredible. I could give you so many illustrations.

I don't understand how anybody could believe in evolution. I don't say that as a preacher, I say that as a human being. Have you ever thought about your body? If you believe in evolution, you've got way more faith than I do. If you believe this machine was an accident, think about it, sir; think about it, ma'am. How could such a finely tuned, magnificent machine be accidental?

One of the things I do in my journey to improved health is read something every day related to health. Sometimes it's just a little statement, sometimes five, ten or fifteen minutes. Not a long time, just something every day.

I want to maximize this body, don't you? It has been created by God. It's a miracle.

What to Do with this Knowledge

So what? Caring for this miraculous body—maximizing its potential—takes immediate and vigilant action. I had to choose to reject procrastination. I had to say, "I've got to do something about this." *Mañana* diet, that was my favorite diet. *Mañana* (in Spanish) means tomorrow. I love that diet, don't you? I was always on the *mañana* diet.

I also love Monday diets. You know the ones: the KFC-on-Sunday-fried-chicken-skin-and-mashed-potatoes-and-gravy splurge, with the justification that, "Tomorrow morning, baby, no more mashed potatoes and gravy for me. My diet is going to kick into high gear after this one last Sunday afternoon fling."

Once I got serious, I knew I had to move on it that day—not on some hypothetical tomorrow. James 4:17 says, "To him who knows to do good and does not do it, to him it is sin." Do you know that it's good to take care of your body? You know it. If you know this, and you're not doing it, this is sin. This was a sin area in my life, and it is something I still struggle with. Why should you improve your health now, not tomorrow? There are many reasons; here are just a few:

You'll Feel Better

You will have more energy and fewer pains; you'll be more alert; you'll be less depressed. Many people struggle with depression. Get your body moving and you'll be shocked at how it lifts your spirits.

You'll Look Better

Do you want to look better and have more confidence? You know that improving your appearance through healthy living will boost it.

You'll Live Longer

Countless studies show that people who are healthy and not significantly overweight live longer than others.

You'll Gain Strength Spiritually

Your body is the temple of God. If you're saved, God lives inside of you. Your body is His temple. If you came into church and somebody had spray painted the walls and messed up the carpets and broken the lights, you'd get mad. I'd get mad too. You'd think, *This is the house of God.*

But the church building isn't the house of God. It is only bricks and mortar, carpet and electrical appliances. What makes it special isn't that it's called a church. What makes the church special is that it is where believers come together. But the building is not His temple.

You are His temple, according to 1 Corinthians 6:19-20: "Or do you not know that your body is the temple of the Holy Spirit who is in you, whom you have from God, and you are not your own? For you were bought at a price; therefore glorify God in your body and in your spirit, which are God's."

When we trash our body-temples, we need to get just as upset about what we're doing as we would if someone trashed our church building. It's time to reject procrastination.

YOUR BODY IS MADE BY GOD AND FOR GOD

Renew Your Mind

You've got to renew your mind. It's time to put off the former things and put on the new things. Ephesians 4:23 says, "Be renewed in the spirit of your mind." You must feed your mind healthy thoughts if you're going to be healthy. Where can you get those?

Read the Bible Every Day
Every day read the Bible. The way to renew your mind is to read it and meditate on what you read.

As you do this, the Holy Spirit will speak to you about specific changes you need to make. Joshua 1:8 says, "This Book of the Law shall not depart from your mouth, but you shall meditate in it day and night, that you may observe to do according to all that is written in it." The only time the word *success* appears in the Bible is in Joshua 1:8. If you're like I am, you want to be a success in life. Since it's important to me and it's only in the Bible once, I want to listen up and hear how God defines it.

You want to measure your success by God's standard, which is obedience to God's commands. Are you observing and doing the Word of God? That's what success is, according to God. Read the Bible every day—and meditate on it. Read it to understand it—not just to get in your obligatory daily allowance. Read it to get to know its Author. This is how to succeed in God's eyes.

Read Health-related Books or Materials Every Day
I'm a busy guy. I don't have time to read lots and lots of stuff. But every day I try to read something to feed my mind a little bit, just to get me thinking about what I need to be thinking about. In 2 Timothy 4:13, Paul asked Timothy to, "Bring the cloak that I left with Carpus at Troas when you come—and the books, especially the parchments." The parchments were God's written Word. Paul also believed in reading other good books.

Every day you ought to spend time reading health-related materials. Remember Hosea 4:6, "My people are destroyed for lack of knowledge." You also may want to listen to health-related teaching. Make a plan to incorporate this material into your life regularly. And stick with it.

Renew that mind, because without that, I think about things I shouldn't think about. I have to renew my mind. I have to get my mind focused on health.

Remember the Benefits

The next way to stay motivated to pursue a *Bod4God* is to remember the benefits. Constantly remind yourself of all the benefits you'll experience. Keep your eye on the prize, because you're going to get hungry. You're going to get lazy. It's a fight. You have to see through that and realize your physical health is going to prosper, and your spiritual health is going to prosper. Keep the benefit before you.

It takes time to change your body. But if you will just say, "God, I'm going to deny myself, and follow You," there is a period where it's tough—but it does get easier. It always will be difficult for me, but it does get better. Your cravings change. When I wake up in the morning, I literally crave a nutritional bar. I crave an apple. That's not what I craved before. Now I crave salads at lunch time. I really crave them; but it wasn't always that way.

Likewise, I crave exercise. Okay, I just exaggerated a little. I like it better than I used to—that much I can say honestly. I can't say I've started craving exercise quite yet. I'm getting there, though; I'm working on it, okay? You need to work through that stuff. Remember the benefits.

As we conclude our thoughts on this subject, I encourage you to pray this prayer:

"Father, I love You, I thank You for Your Word today. Thank You that You can motivate me. Thank You for the truths I've learned today. Whatever area that I need to change, maybe weight, maybe something totally different, use these principles to help me. Lord, open up the key to a better life to me through motivation. In Jesus' name, amen."

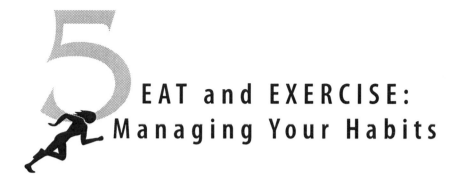

EAT and EXERCISE: Managing Your Habits

*That each of you should know how to possess his own vessel in
sanctification and honor.*
(1 Thess. 4:4)

As we've discussed more than once in this book, the very foundation of building a healthy lifestyle is to realize that God gave you
life, and you're to take your life and your body and please Him in
the things that you do with them. Since there are so many mentions of the word *body* in the Bible, we can know for sure that God
didn't leave us on this earth without direction as to how we should
manage our bodies. You'll hear these things in different venues, but
for me, this literally comes from my heart to your heart.

We can all do better. We can all improve. And maybe your issue isn't weight. Maybe it's something else. I guarantee that if you
take these four keys from our D-I-E-T acrostic and apply them to
that area you are trying to improve, you can make it happen. These
things can work in any area of change that you're trying to imple-
ment in your life. I just happen to be applying these to weight, but
you can use them in other areas.

In this chapter we're going to look at Eat and Exercise. I knew
if I was going to get healthy, I was going to have to manage my
habits better than I had been. I was going to have to bring my
habits under control.

THE BOD 4 GOD
D.I.E.T. PLAN

Dedication: Honoring God With Your Body
Inspiration: Motivating Yourself For Change
Eat & Exercise: Managing Your Habits
T

Again, as I started this process of losing weight, I asked God to give me a passage of Scripture that would be my marching orders, if you will, for this new journey I was going to take. And God burned into my heart Matthew 16:24-25. Here Jesus said to His disciples, "If anyone desires to come after Me, let him deny himself, and take up his cross, and follow Me. For whoever desires to save his life will lose it, but whoever loses his life for My sake will find it." Jesus taught me what I needed to get healthy right here in this passage. He taught me that if I wanted to live, I had to lose, I had to be a loser. That's where I came up with the concept of losing to live.

Jesus said that if you are going to go into this type of journey, you have to deal with self. You have to deny yourself. Self wants to eat things that aren't healthy. Self doesn't want to exercise. Jesus said you have to deny yourself if you want to live, *really* live.

Just like Jesus prayed in Gethsemane to do the Father's will and not take the easy way out, so also Paul acknowledged in 1 Corinthians 15:31, "I die daily." The same is true for us if we really want to fulfill God's will for our lives. We have to die to self.

Jesus said when you do that, you will live. He says if you try to save your life, and you just live for yourself, which so many people do, unfortunately, you're going to lose your life. What that means is your life is going to amount to nothing of eternal consequence and eternal significance. If you want to live an eternally significant life, and not just try to pursue worldly success, if you want to live a significant life, a life where there's a legacy, and a life where you have an eternal impact, lose your life. Give your life to Him. And

Jesus said when you do that, then you'll really live. This portion of Scripture has become my marching order. This has become my lifestyle, and I hope it will affect your lifestyle as well.

Now let's turn our attention to the issue of managing our habits. The main verse that has helped me here is 1 Thessalonians 4:4, where Paul writes: "That each of you should know how to possess his own vessel in sanctification and honor." I had to learn how to possess my body. I had to learn how to manage my body so it was one of holiness and sanctification–one that honored God.

If I was going to lose the weight, if I was going to live healthy, I had to gain control of my body. I had to manage my habits, particularly in the area of eating and exercising. This verse has been a help to me regarding controlling my body, rather than my body controlling me.

Let me share with you some other helpful things.

Obey the Bible

If you're going to manage your habits, you have to understand this is an issue of obedience, or disobedience, according to the Word of God. We have to obey the Bible. This is huge for me, bringing together my belief and my behavior. I always believed I *should* do it, I just didn't behave that way.

The Bible says in Proverbs 4:20-22, "My son, give attention to my words; incline your ear to my sayings. Do not let them depart from your eyes; keep them in the midst of your heart; For they are life to those who find them, and health to all their flesh."

The Bible says if we will follow the Word of God and listen to the Word of God, we will have life and have health. The Bible tells us how to be healthy. There are two basic things taught in the Word of God, and if you obey them, you will lose weight, or you will live a healthy lifestyle.

Number one, you have to eat in moderation. For me—and for many of us who are overweight—that means eating less. For all of us it means to make healthier eating choices. For someone who is anorexic, that will mean eating sensibly, the right things in the

A Bod4God Close-up:
Bobby and Stacy Vickers

How does a chef approach weight loss? With recipes, of course. Bobby Vickers is a hotel chef. He and his wife Stacy are long-time members of Capital Baptist Church.

As team leaders in the Losing to Live competition, the Vickers gave their team recipes for tasty, healthy foods. Things like salads and wraps with beef or chicken and lots of healthy veggies prepared with creative seasonings and spices to make them palate-pleasers.

Bobby and Stacy made a number of small changes to their habits—like giving up soda and substituting frozen grapes for ice cream. They attend Body & Soul exercise class at the church, which they describe as a great program that makes "exercise tolerable" because of its focus on God-centered, uplifting music.

The Vickers are intentional about their food choices, planning their menus ahead at the beginning of each week. "I'm a school teacher," Stacy says. "I keep salads ready—pre-packed in takeout containers with the chicken and dressing separated out." At night when both are too tired to cook complex recipes, "our standby is an omelet," they say.

Eating "adventuresome" recipes created with good health and eating habits in mind has paid big dividends to the couple. He lost thirty-seven pounds, and she lost twenty-one.

right portions to keep their bodies healthy. The Bible also says we need to get the right amount of exercise.

This is especially important for us overweight people to hear. Because one of the excuses we use is metabolism. You see, this is how many of us overweight people think: "I just have a slow metabolism." That's probably true. Some of you are thin, but you know what? You're sinning because you're a glutton. You think you're healthy because you're skinny, but you have a quick metabolism.

You thought you were going to get out of applying this message, didn't you? Many overweight people envy you. We wish we could be like you. We wish we could eat like you do and look like you do. But most of us can't.

I'm neither a scientist nor a nutritionist, but the fact is we must not use a slow metabolism as an excuse to be overweight. If you put less in your mouth, and you get your body moving, you're almost always going to lose weight.

Eat Less

Again, it doesn't matter what your metabolism is, if you put less in your mouth and get moving, the pounds are going to drop. And you folks who have that awesome metabolism that lets you eat like a hog and stay skinny, the Bible still tells you not to overeat.

The Bible mentions many different kinds of foods. That's yet another fact that tells me I have an awesome God. Remember, He created taste buds, and He created food. He is one cool God. Consider the fact that He would give us taste buds and create food for us to enjoy. Wow! You see, God created food, and He wants us to enjoy our food.

I know this is true because of the passage in Deuteronomy 8:7-8, "For the LORD your God is bringing you into a good land, a land of brooks of water, of fountains and springs, that flow out of valleys and hills; a land of wheat and barley, of vines and fig trees and pomegranates, a land of olive oil and honey."

The children of Israel were going into the Promised Land and God wanted them to know what it was going to be like there. He knew they were going to want to know about the food in the Promised Land.

God told them, "Get ready! You're going to love it. There's going to be lots of clean, fresh water. It's going to spring up from deep springs. It's going to flow down from the mountains." Thank God for water. Water is important. *Thank You, God, for rain. Bless*

A BOD4GOD RECIPE BONUS:
Healthy Wraps

The great thing about wraps is that they are creative, individual, and versatile. For a great wrap, create a combination of the following components:

Tortillas (flour, whole wheat, tomato, spinach, roasted garlic) Lean meat (turkey, roast beef, roasted chicken, grilled chicken, tuna, spicy shrimp, even leftover steak from last night's barbecue)
Salad greens or vegetables (lettuce, olives, salsa)
Low-fat dressing (low-fat ranch, chipotle ranch, blue cheese, balsamic vinaigrette)
Low-fat cheese (cheddar, jalapeno jack, provolone)

Procedure:
1. *Spread salad dressing on tortilla. (Steam, microwave or heat so the tortilla wrap becomes soft for easy rolling.)*
2. *Layer lean meat, cheese, and vegetables; then roll tightly. Cut on the bias and serve with a low fat side dish (vinegar slaw, roasted vegetable salad, low-fat grain salad).*

Recipe courtesy of Chef Bobby Vickers, CEC, CCA, CFBE

you, Father, for being Jehovah Jirah, the God who provides rain so we can drink what we need and take care of our bodies.

But that's not all. "You're going to go over to the land I've promised you, and there's going to be wheat, barley, and vines. There are going to be fig trees, pomegranates, olive oil, honey." He's telling them, "Get ready, the food is going to be great!" God wants us to enjoy our food. But the difference is that He invites us to eat to live, not live to eat.

YOUR BODY IS MADE BY GOD AND FOR GOD

He is saying today, "I want you to eat and drink to My glory. When you come to the table, and you sit down for your meal, I want you to use that as a time to glorify Me." This is consistent with 1 Corinthians 10:31, "Whether you eat or drink, or whatever you do, do all to the glory of God."

The last time you went to church you probably walked in thinking, "I'm going to church. I'm going to worship and glorify God." Wonderful. In the same way, when you go to lunch, glorify God.

How do you eat and drink to the glory of God? That's an interesting question. I don't have all the answers except for this: I know you can't overeat and do it to the glory of God. During a radio interview I was asked, "Pastor, what would Jesus eat?" It caught me off guard. I wasn't ready for that question. I thought, *What would Jesus eat?*

Here's how I answered: Number one, Jesus wouldn't be a vegetarian. There's nothing wrong with being a vegetarian. That's a healthy way to eat; it's a great way to eat. Enjoy your veggie burgers, and more power to you. I'm all for you. It's a healthy lifestyle, but I'm going to eat my meat. Jesus ate meat. So we know He wasn't a vegetarian.

Number two, I don't think He would overeat. As we saw earlier, the Bible says if you're a person given to appetite, you ought to take drastic means to change. You ought to take it seriously. You ought to do something about it. And so we need to eat less, and eat better. Not just eat less, but eat healthier.

Drink More Water

You have to drink a lot of pure water to be healthy and lose weight. It is fair to say that every weight loss plan advocates drinking water.

Dr. Don Colbert, MD, in his book *The Seven Pillars of Health* says "Water is the single most important nutrient for our bodies. It is involved in every function of our bodies." Dr. Colbert continues with an explanation about how much water to drink. He says, "Take your weight in pounds and divide it by two. The result is how many ounces of water you should drink daily."

Many people tell me they do not like to drink water. I was the same way. However, as I began to drink more water, I began to like it more and more to the point now that I now crave it. I urge you to discipline yourself to drink more water, and you will see a big difference in your fitness.

Exercise More

God made you to be physically active. When God created man in Genesis 2, does the Bible say the Lord God took the man and put him in the Garden of Eden to sit around and do nothing? No. In Genesis 2:15, "The LORD God took the man and put him in the garden of Eden to tend and keep it." What was God telling Adam? "You've got to be busy, Adam. I'm going to put you in this garden. I want you to maintain it. I want you to be physically active."

Also, right after man sinned, God indicated that He wanted us to be active. As God was sending Adam and Eve from the Garden of Eden, He said, "In the sweat of your face you shall eat bread" (Gen. 3:19a).

So both before and after mankind's fall, from the beginning, God expected man to be physically active.

In the last 100 years, times have changed. We've gone from being an agricultural society to an industrial society to a technological society. There was a time when most people kept the garden and tilled the ground. It was an agricultural society.

There are probably only a few farmers reading this book. I know this because most of the people populating the western world today aren't farmers. Most of us are in the technological side of the culture rather than doing jobs that require physical activity. Of course it's okay to do this type of work, but what it forces us to do is be more intentional when it comes to exercise. Most of us are going to make a living behind a desk or behind a computer and we're not going to get the exercise we need in our jobs. So we have to be more intentional in moving our bodies and getting active. The bottom line is most of us need to schedule physical activity into our lives or we won't get it.

There's only one verse in the Bible that mentions the word *exercise*. The Greek word *gumnasia,* which we translate as *exercise* is mentioned only in 1 Timothy 4:8, when Paul writes, "For bodily exercise profits a little." I loved this verse for years. If anybody talked about exercise, this was one of my memory verses. I would say, "Yeah, that's great, but it only profits a little."

Let me tell you about that verse. It's a comparative statement. It's comparing physical exercise with spiritual exercise. When we exercise physically, we're only taking care of the temporal. When we exercise spiritually, we're taking care of the eternal. Some of you are out of balance in this area. Some of you are physically active and in perfect shape, but you never read your Bible, you don't ever pray, you don't come to church the way you should. You don't exercise yourself spiritually.

Yes, you've got the abs, and you've got the biceps to prove that you're strong in exercise, but let me tell you something. You are going to die one day. You'd better invest yourself in something that's going to outlast you, something of eternal significance. That's what the verse is teaching us. We can't use that verse as an excuse not to exercise because God has told us to be physically active. So we have to be more intentional.

By the way, Paul doesn't tell Timothy that physical exercise doesn't profit anything. What he does say is that it profits little compared to the spiritual.

But they were living in a different day, with different requirements. In those times people were physically active. They walked nearly everywhere they went. They didn't drive a car. They didn't travel by plane. When Jesus said to Lazarus, "Let's go see Mary and Martha," they probably would walk to their house, even though it might be many miles away.

Paul didn't say to Barnabas, "Let's go down to the gym. I need to work out and get on the treadmill." Life was a treadmill!

We have several personal trainers in our church, but there wouldn't have been a need for them back in New Testament times. They wouldn't have had jobs back then, but they have jobs today because of our society.

Body & Soul

Our church partners with a ministry called Body & Soul to offer an awesome exercise program that provides cardio and strength training fitness, set to contemporary Christian music. Body & Soul was developed by fitness specialists Jeannie and Roy Blocher in Germantown, Maryland (www.bodyandsoul.org).

This ministry equips fitness-minded Christians to lead exercise classes both in the church and the community. They also provide an encouraging environment for Christians to improve health and invite their non-Christian friends to do the same.

I recommend that other churches and groups establish this program for their people. Jeannie Blocher gives this great advice, "Develop an exercise program that motivates you to do it day after day. You want to wake up each day saying,

> 'I can do that again today' about your exercise program. What mode of exercise will work for you? We can all find some mode of exercise that will fit into our lives. The most important thing about exercise is not what you do, but that you *do* it!

- If you love the outdoors, walk, jog, bike, hike, or Roller-blade™.
- If you want to pamper your joints and don't mind the water, swim.
- Try group fitness classes, especially faith-based ones like Body & Soul Fitness Ministries where you can find a safe, caring environment, whether you are a beginner or veteran exerciser.
- If you like competition, go for team sports—basketball, soccer, or local softball teams.
- Have a family powwow to decide how each member is going to participate in fitness.
- Plant the value of fitness in your kids at an early age and it will always be a part of their lifestyles.
- Plan active vacations where you build time away around physical activity."

Set a Goal

Next, you have to have a goal—in fact you need two kinds of goals: goals of output and goals of input. Let me explain what I mean: I set out to lose 100 pounds. That was my goal of output. But to reach my goal of output, I had to have a goal of input. I had to drink the water I was supposed to drink. I had to exercise at least three times a week. And the list went on. These were my goals of input.

You have to set goals of input which will lead you to achieve your goal of output.

Additionally, it helps to recognize as you set your goal of output that this is a statement of faith in God. When you state your goal, you have what I call "say it faith." Jesus talked about faith where you say unto this mountain, "Be thou removed" (Matt. 21:21 KJV). It's a vision of a healthier future. You're painting a vision of what you want your life to look like.

In Habakkuk 2:2, God instructs the prophet, "Write the vision. And make it plain on tablets, that he may run who reads it." In other words, keep your goal in front of you.

Write down your weight goal, and keep it in a place where you will see it.

What's in a Goal?

As you create your goal of output, you'll want to be sure it is:

1. *Specific.* "I want to lose some weight" isn't a specific goal. Set a target amount of weight to lose and a reasonable timetable to reach that goal.
2. *Achievable.* The average person is going to lose about one to two pounds a week. If you are really heavy, like I was, you may lose weight faster than that. But slowly and surely you'll most likely move into a phase where you lose about one to two pounds a week. That's what you should expect. So when you're thinking about whether your goal is achievable, you've got to think in those terms.

3. *Measurable.* The thing about losing weight is you can stand on a scale, and you can measure what you're doing.

Choose a Plan that is Best for You

Remember, if you fail to plan, you plan to fail. You can have all the goals in the world, but if you don't have a plan to reach them, you'll never reach your goals. Let me spend the remainder of this chapter helping you discover and create a feasible plan to achieve whatever goal God places on your heart.

You've got to find a plan that fits you. This is so important. My wife and I, for example, do not have the same plan. She's on a shake, meal, shake plan. She's losing weight, and she's getting healthy. I'm proud of her. But what works for her isn't going to work for me. I'm not satisfied drinking a ground-up shake for a meal. I'll tell you this: Steve Reynolds is not going to be grinding anything. I had to find what works for me. You have to find what works for you. (If you're really interested in my eating plan, read on to Chapter 8, where I answer the top ten questions I've been asked about my weight loss.)

James 1:5 says, "If any of you lacks wisdom, let him ask of God, who gives to all liberally and without reproach, and it will be given to him." This reminds us that whenever we are in a quandary, we can ask God for wisdom. I'd challenge you to do that as you create a plan to achieve your goal: Ask God to lead you.

I've had many phone calls from people who want me to endorse their weight-loss or health products. But I believe there are many different ways to lose weight. I'd encourage you to be suspicious of anyone who tells you, "This is the only way." I believe there are many ways to do it. Studies show the key to losing weight is *adherence* to an effective plan. Just ask God to lead you to the right way for you.

Get a Multitude of Counsel

Start talking to people and figuring out all kinds of different options, so you can figure out what will work for you. Listen to what's worked for them. Consider how to adapt their programs for your specific concerns and needs. Get input from lots of sources on your plan. This is a biblical concept as well. Proverbs 15:22 says, "Without counsel, plans go awry, but in the multitude of counselors they are established."

Don't Wait to Make Your Plan; Do it Now

Advance decision-making is critical to a healthy lifestyle. Yet another Proverb has really helped me here: "A prudent man foresees evil and hides himself, but the simple pass on and are punished" (Prov. 22:3). Healthy living requires foresight.

I am busy, like many of you. I have to think about when I am going to exercise—I have to set a plan. If I don't foresee it and plan for it, it doesn't happen.

I went away to a pastors' conference. I knew I was going to be at a nice, fancy hotel. I knew there would be all kinds of good food. I can't say I was perfect, but I did pretty well. Part of the reason I did pretty well is I knew I was going to be breaking my routine. I was going to be in a different setting, and I had to think, *You're going to be down there, you've got to think about how you're going to deal with those potatoes when they're put in front of you. What are you going to do with them?* I gave them away. And the people beside me gave me their salads. What a great deal. I got their salad and they got the potatoes!

Follow a Routine

When you start making changes, your body will probably resist change at first. But if you get on a routine, your body will get used to it.

Rich Kay, in his book, *How I Lost Over 75 Pounds And You Can Too*...offers a piece of helpful information about getting started. He wrote, "I just made some small, simple, changes to start off with that gave me incredible energy and motivation to continue on to my goal." Remember, "small, simple, changes" is great advice to follow when you begin your journey to getting a new body.

We need more of a focus on exercise routines. And walking needs to be a big part of it. Walking is a great way to exercise because it only requires a good pair of walking shoes and you can do it in a lot of places.

Think about the law of sowing and reaping in relationship to your health. The Bible says if you sow to your flesh, you will reap corruption. If you sow to your flesh, eat what you want to eat, and don't exercise, you're going to corrupt your body. But if you sow to the Spirit, you will reap what? Life. Galatians 6:9 encourages us by saying, "Let us not grow weary while doing good, for in due season we shall reap if we do not lose heart."

This is important because when you start out, it's hard. Those first days and weeks are difficult times. But you can find encouragement in this fact: repetition will train your body to perform new habits and crave new things. If you will hang in there, you can train your body.

I love 1 Corinthians 9:27 where Paul says, "But I discipline my body and bring it into subjection, lest, when I have preached to others, I myself should become disqualified." I have to train my body. If I train my body, the good news is that many of the unhealthy things I used to crave I no longer crave.

For example, when I woke up this morning, the first thing I craved was an apple and water. That's literally the first thing I wanted. It hasn't always been that way. Around lunchtime I craved a salad. I wanted a salad because six out of seven days a week I eat a grilled chicken salad. That's pretty much what I eat every lunch. I start thinking about it late in the morning and can't wait to get my salad.

Now I'm a boring person. Understand that my whole routine is totally boring. Most of you would never make it on my plan, because I'm not high maintenance when it comes to all these things. I can pretty much fall into a routine and enjoy it. That's how I'm wired.

You've got to find what works for you, because you're different. I really don't have a sweet tooth. I'm not saying I don't like anything sweet. But when you look at my body, especially before

I began my *Bod4God* quest, it was more about meat and potatoes than cookies. Well, there was a lot of ice cream in there, I will have to admit that.

See if you can fill out the following plan, to be more committed to your own lifestyle changes.

MY BOD4GOD LIFESTYLE PLAN

*Then said Jesus unto his disciples, "If any man will come after me,
let him deny himself, and take up his cross, and follow me. For
whosoever will save his life shall lose it: and whosoever will lose
his life for my sake shall find it."*
(Matt. 16:24-25)

My Eating Plan:

My Exercise Plan:

Prepare for Temptation

Be aware that temptation is going to come. Jesus said to "watch and pray" (Matt. 26:41). How do you do that? One way is to take control of your environment. Romans 13:14 says, "Make no provision for the flesh." What does that mean? That means if you don't bring the potato chip bag in the house, you're not going to eat the potato chips. When you load that cart at the store, you're preparing yourself for home. So if you don't put it in the cart and take it home, it won't be there. Wow, glory to God! But if you take that potato chip bag and put it in there, I guarantee you're providing for your flesh, and you're probably going to sit down and eat the whole bag.

I'm not going to provide for my flesh. Instead, I'm going to let the Holy Spirit take control of me, as you should as well.

As we close out this area of letting God be glorified by our eating and exercising, I invite you to pray:

> *"Father, I love You, and thank You so much for Your Word. Thank You that You can help me have new habits. Show me the goals You have for me. Show me the plans I should establish toward achieving those goals. And give me the strength and tenacity to stick with those plans, even when my body fights against me. In Jesus' name, Amen."*

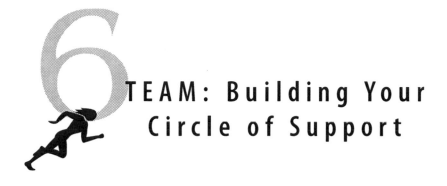

TEAM: Building Your Circle of Support

Iron sharpeneth iron; so a man sharpeneth the countenance of his friend.
(Prov. 27:17 KJV)

Now we're going to turn our attention to the fourth key to having a better body, and that is creating our team support system. You must build your circle of support.

This may be the most important chapter in this book, because it involves getting the people in your life on board with you in your effort to become more healthy.

You know, the biggest room in the world is the room for self-improvement. All of us, I hope, in prayer, are trying to do something better in our lives. You can move these four keys from our D-I-E-T acrostic into that area, and I guarantee they will help you to fulfill your dreams in whatever area you're working on in your life.

T Stands for Team

In every chapter I'm giving you the primary verse that helped me in that particular area of having a *Bod4God*. Today, the key we're talking about is Team: Building Your Circle of Support. The Bible says in Proverbs 27:17, "As iron sharpens iron, so a man sharpens the countenance of his friend."

I understood the impact that people had on me. I learned this spiritually many years ago. My senior year of high school, I made one of the most difficult decisions of my Christian life, and that was to move away from the influence of certain friends. They were good friends in a lot of ways. We grew up together; we were close. I'm not trying to blame them, but they were influencing me in ways that weren't so good. So I made a choice to release those relationships to build new relationships.

That decision took me to a new level spiritually. As I was thinking about this *Bod4God* journey physically, I realized I had to look at my relationships here as well. The same principle that applies spiritually also applies physically. I discovered that I had to find some people who would sharpen me physically and help me.

That meant I had to have a team. I had to build a circle of support. Let me walk you through this whole process of building a circle of support. There were three primary steps I took in building a circle of support.

THE BOD 4 GOD
D.I.E.T. PLAN

Dedication: Honoring God With Your Body
Inspiration: Motivating Yourself For Change
Eat & Exercise: Managing Your Habits
Team: Building Your Circle Of Support

Understand the Value of Team

First I had to understand the value of a team. You have to understand the value of your team. This is important particularly to us men. Ladies, ignore us for a second. I want to talk to the guys for a moment.

Guys, we think we don't need anybody. That's how guys are wired. We're self-made. When there's a marriage problem, you know which partner calls me most of the time? The wife. She is willing to reach out and say, "I need a bigger support system, and maybe, Pastor, you could help me."

Guys, unfortunately we get embarrassed to ask for help, and we say, "I can do it myself." That's the struggle I faced in my life when it came to building a circle of support. I had to realize I couldn't do it alone. Getting healthy usually requires a team effort. You can't be a Lone Ranger. You've got to bring people on board with you.

That shouldn't surprise us, because fellowship and food go together, don't they? When you're fellowshipping with people in our culture, food is usually part of the fellowship.

I know if I want to get people to a meeting, I must have some food. Food always helps people to get to the meeting because that's how our culture is designed. That's a fact.

So I realized I had to get my relationships on board. I had to talk with my wife, and get her on board. I asked her to do this together with me. I had to talk to my children and get them on board with what we were trying to do. I had to talk to co-workers. I had to talk to friends. I even had to talk to my mother. I had to build a circle of support for my newfound journey to a healthy lifestyle.

This journey took an unexpected turn when I discovered the importance of the local church being part of my team. The local church is something I'm giving my life for. The local church is an awesome gift from God. Hebrews 10:24 says, "Let us consider one another in order to stir up love and good works." We are like a team. We ought to consider each other. We shouldn't just think about ourselves, but we ought to think about one another, and we ought to provoke one another to love and to good works. Teamwork is one of the benefits of being part of a local body.

The next verse in Hebrews (10:25) says we shouldn't "forsake the assembling of ourselves together." We ought to attend church as often as possible. When we come, do you know what we ought to be doing? We ought to come with a heart to encourage others. God burdened my heart to make sure our church was a place where people could team up with each other and get more healthy.

Why shouldn't the local church be like this? Why should this be an anomaly? Ecclesiastes 4:9-12 says,

A BOD4GOD CLOSE-UP:
Team Rutabaga

Roota-roota-roota-baga! The chants can be heard across Capital Baptist Church's sanctuary every Sunday evening during the Losing to Live competition. It's the loudest group—and boasts three of the top ten losers. In twenty weeks the team lost a combined 297 pounds. Members credit the enthusiasm of team leader Patricia Dutchie—a self-described dynamo—for their success. She keeps tabs on her team with motivational e-mails and prayer support. The group's prayer list is long—and each member's concerns receive special attention from teammates.

Team member Diane Cornell, one of the biggest losers at forty-one pounds and counting, credits the balance between Bible study, accountability, and Patricia's cajoling as contributors to her loss. Diane shared how that when her granddaughters were with her, "They'd say, 'Grandma, did you learn your verses?' We'd learn them together."

The spiritual aspects of the program have been especially meaningful to Diane, who describes her morning routine as, "I'd eat my oatmeal, drink my water, do my Bible study, and pray for the group. And...the weight just came off!"

Two are better than one, Because they have a good reward for their labor. For if they fall, one will lift up his companion. But woe to him who is alone when he falls, For he has no one to help him up. Again, if two lie down together, they will keep warm; But how can one be warm alone? Though one may be overpowered by another, two can withstand him. And a threefold cord is not quickly broken.

Why is it always better to team up? The passage gives three reasons:

- Teamwork produces mutual *success*. You can have a good reward for your labor.

- Teamwork also produces mutual *support*. When one falls down, the other can lift up his fellow.
- Teamwork produces mutual *strength*. It says that if one prevails against him, two shall withstand him, and a threefold cord is not quickly broken.

There are all kinds of benefits to teamwork: success, support, and strength. TEAM could stand for: Together Everyone Achieves More. If we can come together, everyone achieves more. I had to get over this male mindset, "I can do this alone." I had to be willing to say, "I need a team. I need a circle of support."

Deal with Naysayers on Your Team

Number two, deal with the negative people on your team. You have to realize there may be people in your life who undermine your journey to be more healthy. You have to be willing to confront this. You have to let the people know in your life, "Hey, I'm serious about what I'm trying to do, and I'm asking for your support."

In Matthew 18:15 Jesus says, "If your brother sins against you, go and tell him his fault between you and him alone." You might have to go to some people and say, "Now, listen, I'm serious about this. I want to get healthier, and I really need your support. I need you to come alongside of me and support me, and not undermine what I'm trying to do."

In Daniel 1 there's an awesome example of confronting someone who undermines your health. Daniel was asked to eat the king's meat and drink the king's wine. The problem with that was that these had been offered to idols. The Bible forbade Daniel from partaking in these things.

So Daniel made a decision that he would not defile himself with a portion of the king's meat, nor with the wine he drank. Daniel resolved, "I'm not going to do it." Daniel 1:8 records, "But Daniel purposed in his heart that he would not defile himself with the portion of the king's delicacies, nor with the wine which he drank; therefore he requested of the chief of the eunuchs that he might not defile himself."

You've got to purpose in your heart. You've got to say, "Listen, I am purposing in my heart that I'm going to be more healthy." Now the king wanted Daniel to be healthy—which was why from his perspective he demanded that Daniel eat the choicest foods from his table. But Daniel knew his health—physical and spiritual—would be negatively affected by taking these into his body.

So Daniel made a request. He went to the king's assistant, the prince of the eunuchs, and he said, "Listen, I don't want to defile myself in this way. So let's do a test. It's all about the king wanting me to be strong, wanting me to eat the best and drink the best. But I can't do it his way." Daniel asked to be allowed to drink water and eat beans and vegetables for ten days. He proposed that at the end of ten days he and the others be examined by the king's men. And at the end of those ten days, they looked better. Their health was better.

The king represented someone negative in Daniel's life. And he had to be willing to have resolve, he had to be willing to make a request, and then he experienced the result of having a better body.

You, too, are going to have to deal with the negative people in your life. Most of them don't mean to be negative. Few people in your life are intentionally out to get you, or are intentionally trying to get you to do things that you don't want to do. But even so, you must confront all of the people who would influence you to eat more and exercise less.

You see, it's all about eating less and exercising more. Who is trying to get you to eat things you shouldn't eat? Name them, and then deal with them by making your desires clear and your boundaries plain.

Then again, some people actually may be jealous—they may not want you to do better. We have to be willing to talk about these things. For people like me who have gone up and down for so many years, who is going to take me seriously? I have tried and failed dozens of times. For most of us who have had trouble in this area, that's our story. Who's going to believe me now when I'm going to do something different?

We have to understand that it's going to take a while, because you reap what you sow. It's going to take a while for people to really get on board with your resolve. But you've got to let them know, "I'm serious about this. I want you to be a part of my circle of support."

My mother likes to express her love by feeding people. I'm like that myself. I enjoy cooking for people. People are going to be like that in our lives, and we have to think that through, and we have to deal with that.

Choose a Top-notch Team

Note that I had to consciously choose wise people for my team. You see, the Bible says, "He who walks with wise men will be wise, but the companion of fools will be destroyed" (Prov. 13:20). I had to choose wise people to be part of my team. I had to find people who would come alongside of me, like Moses in Exodus 17:12, where it says his "hands became heavy." Every time he held up his hands and stood for God, his team won. But when his team lost, it was because his arms were heavy and he couldn't hold up his hands. So he had Aaron and Hur help him hold up his arms.

I had to bring some Aarons and Hurs into my life to physically help me, and there were three categories of people I chose.

People Who Will Educate You

You've got to become a student of health. You've got to read; you've got to study; you've got to talk to people; you've got to talk to your doctor. My doctor played a major role in my weight loss and was always there to ask me how was I doing, how was my eating and exercising. For a long time I didn't give him a good answer or have any good news to report to him. Although he was kind, he didn't back down.

I was diabetic, and I was supposed to go to the doctor a lot. I didn't go to the doctor a lot. You know why? Because I didn't want to hear what I should be doing (and wasn't doing) from the doctor, over and over again. Maybe you can relate to that. But he didn't back down when I told him I was not exercising.

When I started exercising, did he tell me I was doing well to exercise three times a week? You know what the man said to me? "You eat every day, why don't you exercise every day?" I had to acknowledge he made a good point.

Authors are among the other people who can educate you. I challenge you to read books, articles, and Web pages written by people who can educate you. There is great information available to us today.

Invest in your health by purchasing books that can help you. Read and study and learn. You've got to get these people on your team.

People are on my team who don't even know me, and I'll probably never meet them this side of heaven. But they are on my team.

People Who Will Encourage You

Next, select people who will encourage you. You need to have role models. As I said earlier, Mike Huckabee, the governor of Arkansas as I write, is my role model. I look to him as a great example. I've seen his life, and I've read his book on how he lost weight, and he's my role model. He's a hero to me. He encourages me.

I've had a lot of people in my church encourage me. You need people who are going to encourage you, people who are going to come alongside you and encourage you to keep pursuing your goals.

Likewise, one of our Losing to Live participants, kindergarten teacher Peggy Ottenheimer, has lost twenty-four pounds. She says, "I have been on a low-fat diet for ten years and didn't lose weight. I joined Curves™ for two years. Still no loss. It wasn't happening."

What does Peggy credit for her success this time? "I needed a group to hold me accountable. It was a combination of things. Dedicating it to God and doing it to God's glory. And providing the extra oomph I needed was the accountability of our whole group behind me."

She says she's become a "walking billboard" for Capital Baptist Church and the program—because every time someone asks her how she lost the weight, she is excited to tell how successful weight loss and healthier living finally happened for her.

People Who Will Equip You
Finally, we all need people who will equip us, who will show us how to do what we've purposed to do. Many people are like I was: they don't exercise. I don't have a personal trainer work with me on a regular basis. I think it would be great to have a regular personal trainer, but I just don't happen to have one. However, the first time I went to the gym to exercise, a personal trainer took me around to show me the machines. He explained how to use each piece of equipment at the gym without injuring myself, what each of them would do to help me, and how to build up my endurance on each apparatus.

That personal trainer had lost over 100 pounds himself. He also told me about the CLIF® BAR, which has been a big help to me. It is an organic bar, and I eat one every morning. And you know what, I may have never known about that, except that I was equipped by that trainer. He helped me.

Additionally, as I've mentioned earlier, we have a program at our church called Body & Soul, and it's an awesome aerobic exercise program. The class leaders of a program like this one can help you to learn how to exercise.

Just like I have, find people who will participate on your team and who will spur you on toward your *Bod4God* commitment. Find some equippers. Find some people who can show you how to do it.

A healthy lifestyle requires you to be a part of a team, rather than a Lone Ranger. It requires you to deal with the negative people in your life and to find wise people to help you. Don't do it alone. Join a team of losers and get healthy for God. Now, let's pray this prayer together.

"Father, I love You, and I thank You for Your Word. Please lead me to people who can assist me in living a more healthy lifestyle. Give me strength and wisdom to properly handle people who are a negative influence. Help me encourage the people around me to take care of their bodies. In Jesus' name, amen."

THE

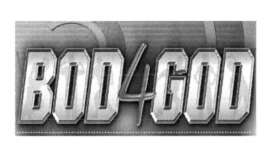

GAME PLAN FOR SUCCESS

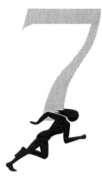

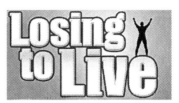

Competition

Restore to me the joy of Your salvation and grant me a willing spirit to sustain me.
(Ps. 51:12)

I've said it before, but it bears repeating—I'm not content to see my own *Bod4God* plans achieved. I want to see a whole church—in fact whole churches—full of *Bod4God* losers. When I preached the *Bod4God: Four Keys to a Better Body* sermon series at Capital Baptist Church, my goal was to motivate our congregation to become the biggest group of losers in the United States.

But a sermon series alone wasn't going to help people get there. So, coinciding with the series, we launched the Losing to Live Weight Loss Competition, as an opportunity to lose weight in a fun, supportive environment. It was a natural outflow of the Team key—I wanted to give others the same kind of team support and motivation I had received from my own group of encouragers.

What I found after experiencing this competition was that the 150 people who joined the competition—a large percent of whom weren't members of our church—became my encouragement, motivation, and inspiration. I felt as if they had come alongside me in making a difference for me, for themselves, and for so many people all around them.

A BOD4GOD CLOSE-UP:
Eric Larsen: Biggest Loser

Six months ago, if you'd told Eric Larsen he'd be the biggest loser—he'd hardly have been proud. In twenty weeks that's exactly what he is—the biggest loser, sporting sixty-six fewer pounds.

"My father had two heart attacks and my mother recently had one heart attack," Eric explains. "I have struggled with my weight since I was thirteen, and I had the worst eating habits you could imagine. I rarely ate a vegetable—I was a meat-and-potatoes guy. And I was into junk food."

What made Eric change his erring ways? "The testimony of Pastor Steve about how he lost the weight. Hearing from someone who was actually doing something about it. That's what reached me." He began with a New Year's resolution—after gorging on chocolate over the holidays. "Now I do Slimfast™ Optima," he says. Why? Because it's chocolate.

One key to his weight loss is a weekly "cheat night," where he uses some restraint, but does allow himself a treat or two.

Another key is a Yahoo e-mail group he's participating in as part of the competition. The group discusses their week's struggles, prayer requests, food tips, even recipes. He says this support has been a lifeline that's kept him moving forward on this new lifestyle. And what about the veggies? The group shared a green-bean salad recipe that has made a veggie convert out of him.

To open the plan up to those outside our congregation (as an outreach and a ministry to them), we advertised on local radio and with brochures and an announcement on the church's marquee. Our materials offered this invitation: "Don't try to lose weight all by yourself. Join a team of losers at Capital Baptist Church."

YOUR BODY IS MADE BY GOD AND FOR GOD

With the media attention from the *Washington Post* and local and national (later, even international) TV, people came in droves to find out what would motivate a Baptist pastor to take such a personal interest in his congregation's physical health. And when Fox News' Neil Cavuto labeled me the "anti-fat pastor," it certainly got people's attention.

We kicked off the competition on Sunday, January 14, 2007, with—of all things—an orientation luncheon. We have a professional chef in our church, Bobby Vickers, and for the luncheon Bobby prepared a beautiful (and delicious) healthy spread. Lots of vegetables and tasty salads along with a "wrap bar" that let participants choose healthy meats and cheeses and veggies to fold into their own personalized soft tortilla wrappers. (See page 60 for some hints from Bobby on creating your own favorite healthy wraps.)

It was a great rah-rah event—and dozens of people found themselves surprised that they were enjoying the healthy fare every bit as much as their old unhealthy choices. It was the first among countless successes experienced by the participants, who lost a total of 1,310 pounds in the program's twenty weeks.

The Evening's Agenda

Each week competitors had the opportunity to weigh-in (in privacy, using a physician's scale that measured Body Mass Index as well as weight) during each of our three Sunday morning services, as well as during our Sunday evening competition group meetings. Many found they preferred weighing in early in the day (before Sunday lunch or dinner), which was just fine with us.

At the big gathering in the church auditorium on Sunday evenings, we'd open by celebrating each team's achievements of the previous week. (By the way, each of the ten teams chose a fruit or vegetable name for themselves. We had lemons and passion fruit, squash and rutabagas, to name a few.) The teams competed for their highest weight loss percentages (Team Rutabaga was consistently among the top three), and individuals on the teams competed to become one of the top ten losers.

Input from Experts

After the cheerleading sessions we invited various experts to be speakers to the whole group. One week, for example, a medical doctor in our congregation, Liz Berbano, gave us an update on the latest medical research on how to overcome obesity. Another week the husband of one of our competitors (who is a certified internist) came on a Sunday morning during weigh-in to offer baseline blood work (glucose, cholesterol, and blood pressure) for the minimal fee of $15 to any competitor who wished to participate.

Another week Vivian Hutson, a registered dietician from our congregation, was our evening's guest speaker. Vivian became key to our program, as she directed the weigh-in of each participant week after week, offering encouragement and challenge wherever needed.

Vivian is a great story. She is a lieutenant colonel in the U.S. Army. She's been involved as a key player in creating our church's health ministry plan—and she's been a real blessing. Her training gives her a unique perspective to offer competitors and the knowledge on how best to motivate them.

Vivian found the weigh-in times were great opportunities to get to know the people and listen to their deeper needs. "They didn't just want to talk about their diets. They'd tell me if they had a stressful week; they would promise to do better," she says. But Vivian was careful never to be judgmental—even when someone had a gainer week. "I ask them what they wish they would have done differently. Then I'd challenge them to put it behind them. That was last week! Now let's make healthy lifestyle choices for this week." And, of course, Vivian would help them focus on God, rather than the stress or unhappiness of the previous week. "We pray about it—to have a healthier body not just for self-gratification, but for God."

Vivian and her team kept the records to update our database each week—her logs helped track individual and team weight loss by pounds, by percentage, and by BMI. She comments, "When I teach other community nutrition classes, I have never seen the success of any program like I see in this program. I think what we see here will last for a long time, because they are doing it for God—for the right reason."

When we didn't have special speakers, we'd often see portions of videos—especially as they related to our small group break out time.

The goal of this first portion was to provide information that would help motivate and equip competitors to move forward with their healthy-lifestyle choices.

Group Time

But the big-group sessions were just the beginning. Most competitors really connected with the program when they broke into their small group teams. There they would go over the week's assigned reading. We used the material from this book and other health-related resources.

This was a non-threatening time to interact with the material, to share ideas on what worked and what didn't work for each individual, to cheer for successes, to encourage where needed, and most of all to pray with each other. The teams built relationships so strong that they prayed for each other all week long—some even used the phone or e-mail to keep the lines of communication open between Sunday evenings.

As the program wound down in June, I heard more than a few competitors wish aloud that they could keep meeting with their teams over the summer—because they attributed their weight-loss success and much of their spiritual growth to their team relationships. For most participants, then, the team time was the highlight of the program.

Exercise Options

In addition to the Sunday evening sessions, Capital Baptist Church opened its doors to competitors and even to those not signed up in the competition for a God-centered exercise program Body & Soul, developed by aerobics and exercise specialists Jeannie and Roy Blocher in Germantown, Maryland.

YOUR BODY IS MADE BY GOD AND FOR GOD

Dr. Liz Berbano became our Body & Soul leader, offering group exercise three times a week with weekday, evening, and weekend options. She loves this program because it contains elements of spiritual and physical exercise in each session. Billed as "cardio and strength training to contemporary Christian music," Body & Soul provides an inspirational, safe, modest setting where active seniors, middle-aged folks, even teens can work out together in a non-threatening environment—while filling their minds with biblical messages.

We had several husband and wife teams doing Body & Soul together, and at least one family, Robert and Caroline Murphy, whose teen boys came week after week to exercise with them. "I joined to encourage my wife and do it with her," Robert says. "Now our two sons Kyle (15) and Michael (16) are doing it with us."

Caroline adds, "Pastor, you talked about team—my strongest support system is my family—they are my team. Since joining the program, we pray more together, we read more together, my husband has us memorizing the book of James together. It is a good foundation for our kids." In twenty weeks Robert lost thirty-four pounds and Caroline lost thirty-nine pounds.

But other participants are finding ways to exercise that better fit their unique lifestyles—and their schedules. Some are swimming or working out at Curves™ or other gym facilities. Sabrina Prime, a wife and mom who has lost thirty-one pounds, joined Bally's gym on a ninety-day free offer coupon that was available when she signed up for the competition. She made such good use of the gym's offerings that she decided to rejoin when the ninety days were up.

And eighty-three-year-old Bob McAllister of our congregation is one of the most active guys in the whole program. He goes to the gym three days a week, works out on the equipment for a half hour before going to aerobics class, then cycles and does other exercises besides. That, combined with eating smaller portions, helped him lose twenty-six pounds in twenty weeks.

A Big Finish!

With such a winning program going on over so many weeks, we wanted to plan a big finale—one that would top our opening luncheon and yet be consistent with all the *Bod4God* progress we'd all made. So we planned a 5K run/walk, which we advertised and opened up to the community. It would be a program wrap-up, a celebration, and a community outreach—all rolled up into one.

The 5K path started and ended on our church property, and we were able to get professional runners to help establish the route. We walked the route several Sunday evenings before the event, and we enlisted volunteers from the congregation to help out along the route on race day. We found a number of corporate sponsors to donate prizes and products for the event, and after a few planning meetings we were ready to run the race.

Finally, when race day came on June 23, 2007, 350 people participated, many of whom were among the 150 Losing to Live competitors and many more of whom were from the community at large. It was an event deemed a success by all.

Competitor Damon Johnson said, "My wife Charlene and I enjoyed the fellowship, running for Jesus against obesity, and the healthy brunch you provided for all of us. Keep on encouraging all God's people to be the best that God wants them to be and inspiring them all to enjoy eating healthy, exercising, and staying faithful to the Lord by doing His will."

But even with the competition over, the lifestyle changes it brought won't soon be forgotten—and weight loss won't soon be regained. Steve Richardson, who participated in the competition along with his wife Mary Jane, says, "I have learned to deal with the emotional part of weight loss. We know how to eat right. We both know about exercise and physical fitness, we have this knowledge, but we have to be motivated by something."

That something, he says, has been the *Bod4God* program. "My thought processes are different now," he says. "I remember praying God, it is in your hands, guide me."

Obviously, God has guided Steve (he's lost forty pounds) and Mary Jane (she's lost twenty-eight pounds)—and the others who have found in the competition the support and motivation to change their lives for God's glory.

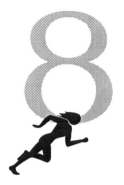

TOP TEN:
Questions
and Answers

*But sanctify the Lord God in your hearts, and always be ready to
give a defense to everyone who asks you a reason for the hope that
is in you, with meekness and fear.*
(1 Pet. 3:15)

As I've done interviews with mass media folks and as I've talked
with *Bod4God* participants one on one, I've been asked a lot of
questions. So what I want to do in this chapter is answer the top
ten questions about *Bod4God*. We'll begin once again in Matthew
16, the passage God has so used in my life to help me seek to have
a *Bod4God*, where Jesus taught us here about losing to live.

Jesus stated that the Christian life means losing to live. He
made this statement six times in the Word of God. The message
was this: if you want to live, you've got to be a loser. What do you
have to lose? You have to lose yourself. You have to deny yourself.
You have to take up Jesus' cross and follow Him. And Jesus said if
you will do that, then you will live. If you really want to live, be a
loser. Lose yourself and live for Him.

As I think about this issue of questions and answers, a verse that
has been on my heart a lot in recent days is 1 Peter 3:15 which says,
"But sanctify the Lord God in your hearts, and always be ready to
give an answer." We're to give a defense (or as the old King James
version put it, an answer) to everyone who asks you a reason for
the hope that is in you. You know, losing to live has created hope
in my life. It's a fire God has ignited in my heart. It's a hope God

has put in my spirit, and God has allowed me an opportunity to share this message. I want to apply that verse to *Bod4God*.

**THE BOD 4 GOD
D.I.E.T. PLAN**

Dedication: Honoring God With Your Body
Inspiration: Motivating Yourself For Change
Eat & Exercise: Managing Your Habits
Team: Building Your Circle Of Support

Question #1: Why are so many Christians overweight?

If being healthy is so important, why do so many Christians struggle in this area and in this way? The truth is, this is an issue among all people, but it is an issue among Christians in particular.

Ken Ferraro, a professor at Purdue University and director of Purdue's Center on Aging and the Life Course, has done a lot of research on certain people groups and weight issues. He posted an article on Purdue's official Web site on August 24, 2006, titled, "Study Finds Some Faithful Less Likely to Pass the Plate." That title is a takeoff on passing the offering plate, but it's talking about Christians' propensity to overeat. Here are a few highlights of that article:

> Religious shepherds need to keep better watch over their flocks and add activities to keep from fattening them up, says a Purdue University researcher who has found that some religious activities may promote obesity.

> America is becoming known as a nation of gluttony and obesity, and churches are a breeding ground for this problem," says Ken Ferraro, a professor of sociology, who has studied religion and bodyweight since the early 1990s. "If religious leaders and organizations neglect this issue, they will contribute to an epidemic that will cost the health care system millions of dollars, and reduce the quality of life for many parishioners.

The reason I like this article so much is because he goes through and looks at different possibilities as to why this is such an issue in the Christian community, and he talks about different possibilities for why this is true. For example, he talks about the fact that this sin of overeating is an accepted sin among Christians. We might preach against other things, but this is something we don't talk about much, and so maybe that's one reason it's a problem in our society, and particularly in the Christian community.

He offers other possible reasons for the problem, as well. But what I like about this so much is that right from the beginning of this article, it puts the blame where the blame needs to go. I believe everything rises and falls on leadership, and I believe the main reason people are overweight in the pews is because pastors are overweight behind the pulpit.

You can blame-shift and blame me. But you can't blame me anymore. You see, pastors struggle with this just like other people struggle with this, and most pastors, myself included, have a difficult time preaching on anything they're not practicing.

In Acts 20:26-27 Paul is preaching to preachers, and he says to them, "Therefore I testify to you this day that I am innocent of the blood of all men. For I have not shunned to declare to you the whole counsel of God." Paul is saying, "Listen, my hands are clean. Your blood is not on my hands. I'm not responsible for you in your bad behavior. I have not shunned, I have not kept from preaching to you *all* the counsel of God."

God tells us in His Word how to manage our bodies. That's part of the counsel of God, and we've neglected this area in the Word of God. Do you know what God says to the pastors? "Take heed, therefore, unto yourselves, and to all the flock, over which the Holy Ghost has made you overseers" (Acts 20:28 KJV). Why? "To feed the church of God." That doesn't mean feed the church of God potluck dinners. We've done a good job of feeding the stomachs of the people in our congregations. But this verse is talking about feeding their souls with the Word of God.

My answer to why so many Christians are overweight is because so many pastors are overweight. So many Christian leaders are overweight, and we have neglected this portion of the Word of God. I have set this horrible example for years. And even those who aren't overweight don't preach against it enough (perhaps for fear of offending major portions of their congregations).

But the good news is that if the problem lies in the pulpit, perhaps the answer lies in the pulpit, too. If God will allow me, and I'm praying He will, I'm going to create a movement throughout this country, and throughout the world trying to get pastors and spiritual leaders on board with having a *Bod4God* and preaching and teaching this to their congregations.

I'm praying that God will use the success of our *Bod4God* program to encourage other churches to start similar programs in their communities.

Question #2: What are your four keys to a better body?

People ask me, "How did you lose weight?" I say, "There are four keys." And the typical response is, "What are the four keys?" You'll recall that I used the acrostic D-I-E-T: Dedication. Inspiration. Eating and Exercise. Team.

Key #1 is Dedication: Honoring God with Your Body
For me it was a matter of bringing together my belief system and my behavior. I realized what the Bible taught, yet my behavior didn't reflect it. So for me, bringing those two together meant dedicating my body to God and honoring Him with my body.

My biggest breakthrough was realizing I needed to depend on God to help me. I couldn't do it alone. I believe some people can lose weight and get healthy without God. There's plenty of evidence to demonstrate this, but I'm not one of them. I needed God to help me.

Galatians 5:16 says, "Walk in the Spirit, and you shall not fulfill the lust of the flesh." I had to learn to incorporate walking in the Spirit not just in the pulpit, but also in improving my health. I had to bring those two together in my life.

A BOD4GOD CLOSE-UP:
Liz Berbano, MD

Capital Baptist Church member Liz Berbano is delighted her church is making such strides toward physical health, alongside spiritual health. It matters to her, especially because she and her husband Darren are medical doctors.

Liz, formerly a lieutenant colonel in the U.S. Army and now a staff physician at Walter Reed Army Medical Center, has done her homework on weight loss and aerobics programs. "A program will work only if there is adherence. JAMA (the Journal of the American Medical Association) says a program has to motivate people to adhere to it."

She quotes a study published in JAMA, "One way to improve dietary adherence rates . . . may be to use a broad spectrum of diet options, to better match individual patient food preferences, lifestyles, and cardiovascular risk profiles."

Liz believes Bod4God is seeing success because it offers healthy eating and exercise options and gives a spiritual reason for adherence—which motivates spiritually minded people.

Liz is the aerobics trainer for the church's Body & Soul program, which she says allows participants to be modest and to participate at various levels of activity. "It's nourishing for the mind and heart, as well as the body," she says about the program that features music rich in biblical content.

Key #2 is Inspiration: Motivating Yourself for Change
How do you get started? How do you stay on track?

You've got to be motivated. You've got to find out what will motivate you to get started with the changes you need. The fact that you are reading this book is a good start.

John 10:10 is the key verse for me in that area where Jesus said, "The thief does not come except to steal, and to kill, and to destroy. I have come that they may have life, and that they may have it more abundantly." The thief, Satan, has an agenda for your life and mine: he comes to steal, and to kill, and to destroy. For many of us, he is using a knife and a fork to do it.

But Jesus says, "I come to give you life." The thing that motivates me is life. I want to live a better life, and I want to live a longer life. And I know if that's going to happen, I've got to live a healthy lifestyle. A healthy life will lead to a better life and, more than likely, a longer life.

A lot of times we want to lose weight for some special event. Maybe there's a high school reunion coming up, or a wedding coming up, or some big family event, and we say, "I've got to lose a few pounds so I'll look good."

That's good, but this is better, because life is as long as you live. It's not like an event that comes and goes, it's something you carry with you all the time. This is my inspiration: I want to live an abundant life both in quality and quantity.

Key #3 is Eat and Exercise: Managing Your Habits
I knew I had to manage my habits. I had to learn 1 Thessalonians 4:4, "That each of you should know how to possess his own vessel." *Vessel* there means body. I had to learn how to possess my body better by improving my habits of eating and exercising, essentially eating less and exercising more.

Key #4 is Team: Building Your Circle of Support
I needed other people. Proverbs 27:17 says, "Iron sharpens iron, so a man sharpens the countenance of his friend." I had to bring people into my life who could sharpen me when it came to better health. I had to bring into my life people who knew things I needed to know about health. I had to allow them to impact my life through books, through one-on-one encounters, through group-type settings, etc.

Those are the four keys to a better body.

YOUR BODY IS MADE BY GOD AND FOR GOD

Question #3: How can I apply these keys to other addictions in my life?

These are transferable concepts. In other words, these keys can apply to other areas of your life besides losing weight.

The Losing to Live message started with a sermon series that took the principle of losing to live and showed how it applies to lots of different areas. We talked about losing debt; we talked about losing anger; we talked about losing lust; we talked about losing stress; and finally, we talked about losing weight. Because you know what? All these problems are based on elevating self above God's Word. When you do that, you will live.

The principles apply. In Galatians 2:20 Paul said, "I have been crucified with Christ; it is no longer I who live, but Christ lives in me." It's about dying to self and letting Christ live in and through you.

Maybe for you it's debt. Debt is usually all about self, buying things you can't afford, and getting yourself in debt. Maybe it's anger, "Oh, you offended me, you did something to me, and I'm going to get angry at you. I have a right to get angry at you." Or lust. "I'm going to look at what I want to look at; I'm going to do what I want to do; I'm going to act the way I want to act." Or stress, "I can get through life all by myself. I don't need God or anyone else to help me." These principles are also about stress.

These principles can be transferred to other areas. For example, by using the acrostic DIET in dealing with financial debt.

D–Dedication. Just start out saying, "God, my money belongs to You. You are the owner of it. I'm going to honor You with my money." I–Inspiration. What could be your inspiration? Life works there, too. Because I'll tell you, if you want a tough life, then get yourself in a heap of debt.

Eat and Exercise: Managing Your Habits. Maybe eat and exercise doesn't specifically apply, but what about managing your habits? Maybe you need to cut up the credit cards. Maybe that's a habit. Team. Our church offers small-group studies designed specifically to team up with other people who struggle in the area of finances and to provide good support and encouragement to get debt under control.

YOUR BODY IS MADE BY GOD AND FOR GOD

Why not team up with some other people and study the Word of God together, as it applies to debt? Build a circle of support for getting your money together.

You see, you can take D-I-E-T and apply it to any one of these areas, and it works.

Question #4–What does the Bible mean when it says your body is the temple of the Holy Spirit?

The Bible says in 1 Corinthians 6:19-20, "Do you not know that your body is the temple of the Holy Spirit who is in you, whom you have from God, and you are not your own? For you were bought at a price; therefore glorify God in your body and in your spirit, which are God's."

I've discovered this is probably the number one passage people use to help them lose weight. As I talk to people, this passage comes up a whole lot. So what does it mean?

It Means God's Spirit is a Resident in Your Life

That Scripture assumes that the moment you came to Christ, the moment you were saved, the Holy Spirit came into your life. Jesus said, "And I will pray the Father, and He will give you another Helper, that He may abide with you forever—the Spirit of truth, whom the world cannot receive, because it neither sees Him nor knows Him; but you know Him, for He dwells with you and will be in you" (John 14:16-17). God lives in you. Think about it, you as a Christian, actually house Deity.

He doesn't live in any church building. There is nothing sacred about a church building except it is a place where we come together to corporately worship the Lord. Our bodies are sacred because they are God's temples.

We're To Reflect the Glory of God

1 Corinthians 6:20 says, "For you are bought with a price, therefore glorify God in your body." Because my body is His temple, I should treat it accordingly.

YOUR BODY IS MADE BY GOD AND FOR GOD

We need to understand that 1 Corinthians 10:31 says, "There-fore, whether you eat or drink, or whatever you do, do all to the glory of God." The Bible tells us one of the ways we can glorify God is through what we eat and what we drink.

Question #5–Does Jesus care whether a person is skinny or fat?

That's quite a question. Now, I'm not talking about, Does Jesus love us? Jesus loves us either way. But you know what? He does care if we're skinny or fat. Let me tell you why I say that.

He Wants us to Live
Do you know He died so that you could live? Did you know that? He is all about you living. The Bible says He gave His precious blood so you could live.

I have never doubted the love of God in my life. He doesn't love me any more today because I've lost weight. But He does care, and He's delighted that I've lost weight, because He knows I can live better, and probably live longer, because of it. He does care.

He was nailed to that cross; He suffered and died on that cross because He wanted us to live for all of eternity with Him. And He wants us to enjoy the journey.

He came to give us an abundant life on this earth, an eternal life in heaven, and He cares.

He's not going to love you any less or any more because you lose weight or don't lose weight. It's not about His love, but He does care.

Question #6–Is overeating a sin?

Yes! It is a sin. The Bible says in 1 Thessalonians 5:23, "Now may the God of peace Himself sanctify you completely; and may your whole spirit, soul, and body be preserved blameless at the coming of our Lord Jesus Christ." God wants to sanctify us wholly—that means our whole spirit and whole body. Part of being sanctified is our eating pattern. So yes, I think the Bible bears out God's perspective that overeating is a sin.

Question #7—What is your eating and exercise plan?

This is a popular question because people always want to know, "What are you eating? What are you doing that's finally helping you lose weight?"

There are many ways to lose weight. I am not all about any one way. I've had lots of people try to get me to adopt things, saying "We've got to come see you, and you've got to tell everybody about our plan." That plan may be wonderful. It probably will work for some people. But I'm not about endorsing any one plan, because I believe you can lose weight lots of different ways.

The problem isn't that we don't have enough plans, the problem is we don't stick to the plans or haven't found the right plan for us. My wife and I are not on the same plan. My wife is losing weight, but she's not losing it the way I'm losing it. Husband and wife. Even we're not on the same page with this thing. We're cool with that. She's excited about what she's doing; it's working for her, and I'm proud of her.

Your breakthrough will come as you seek out a plan that works for you.

My Food Intake

What's working for me is kind of a low carb-type deal, I guess, if you had to classify it. I'm eating some certain carbs. Now it's also boring. I'm a boring guy. I don't have to have a lot of variety of foods in my life, at least not while I'm in this season of life.

A lot of you are different in that way. You've got to come up with all kinds of things, and you get your cookbooks out, and you make this, and you make that, and you're on the thirty-minute meals and all that stuff. I'm not that way.

Here's what I've begun doing pretty much every day since I embarked on my weight-loss journey. I start my day by eating a nutritional bar. My favorite is the CLIF® BAR.

This bar is very nutritious, and I like it a lot. I'll eat one, or some-times two, a day. I eat an apple, sometimes two a day.

With breakfast I drink thirty-two ounces of water, and yes, I also drink coffee. I'm putting everything down here. This is full disclosure. My day off I'll fix eggs sometimes. On Wednesday we have our staff meeting, and somebody fixes us eggs. I will typically eat those. So I vary in those couple of situations for breakfast. But on a typical day that's what I do.

For lunch I get a grilled chicken salad and low-fat dressing, and water. If I go out to eat, that's what I'll order. A lot of times I'll just go to a fast-food place and pick up different ones. Pretty much everybody has one. On my day off I'll make one. See, I make the best you've ever had; they're delicious.

Then I have a snack at late afternoon, an early evening snack. A lot of times this will be the second bar or second piece of fruit and coffee.

For dinner I have lean meat, and five out of seven days a week, chicken. I have green vegetables like broccoli or green beans and diet soda. Yes, I know, diet soda. Then I have some fruit. A lot of times I'll have an orange at night, or grapes, or something like that.

Each Friday night is my cheat night. The longer I go, the less I need cheat night, but particularly in the beginning it was the most wonderful day in all the world. I funnel my cravings into cheat night. If I was craving ice cream, I'd think, *Just two more days and Friday night you can go get your ice cream and have the greatest time of your life.* Literally, the longer I go, the less I need this fix.

I am on a lifestyle plan, and what that means is if it's a very special event (now, don't try to find a special event every day!) —I mean something special, like Christmas Day—I will eat my Christmas meal. I had a good time Christmas Day. I plan to do this the rest of my life, and on my plan for Christmas Day you eat the Christmas meal.

So periodically, there is a special event, and I will partake of the special event—while watching my portions carefully.

YOUR BODY IS MADE BY GOD AND *FOR* GOD

My Exercise Plan

I started out very slow. The biggest mistake people make in exercise is to overdo it when they first start out. I am slowly building up my routine. Today I do forty-five minutes on the treadmill, and fifteen different weightlifting activities three times a week. It works for me. I didn't get that out of a book; I didn't get it from somebody's plan. I just started doing this stuff; I started liking it; I kept on doing it; and I kept on losing weight.

But again, you don't have to do this. Find something that works for you. But stick to it.

Question #8–How should I respond when tempted to do unhealthy things?

We talked about that earlier. But one of the biggest things is disciplining your mind, because what you allow yourself to think about is what you do, and what you do is what you feel. If you want to change your feelings, change your doing. If you want to change your doing, change your thinking.

Everything I've ever eaten started right in my mind. I said, "Whoa, nice, very nice." And then I ate it. And then I felt bad. So if I want to feel better, I've got to *do* better. If I'm going to do better, I've got to think better. "Casting down arguments and every high thing that exalts itself against the knowledge of God, bringing every thought into captivity to the obedience of Christ." (2 Cor. 10:5).

The Bible says when I think of that big Hershey's chocolate bar with almonds, I've got to cast down that imagination. I've got to bring every thought into obedience to Christ.

One of the things that helps me a lot is Galatians 6:7-8, "Do not be deceived, God is not mocked; for whatever a man sows, that he will also reap. For he who sows to his flesh will of the flesh reap corruption, but he who sows to the Spirit will of the Spirit reap everlasting life." Do you want corruption or life? I want life. So I think a lot about life and that begins to change my feelings and my doing.

YOUR BODY IS MADE BY GOD AND FOR GOD

Question #9–What can I do about overeating because of the stress in my life?

A lot of people eat for comfort. They're under a lot of stress, and so they eat. I've told you earlier, a lot of us who come from the South associate high-fat, rich foods with comfort. It's what we grew up with. It's comforting to us to eat these things.

But the Bible calls us to turn to Christ rather than to food. Philippians 4:6-7 says, "Be anxious for nothing, but in everything by prayer and supplication, with thanksgiving, let your requests be made known to God; and the peace of God, which surpasses all understanding, will guard your hearts and minds through Christ Jesus."

There is a direct correlation between prayer and peace. And that's peace, not piece. Make sure you get the spelling right. What can I do about overeating because of the stress in my life? Turn to Christ rather than to food.

Question #10–Why does the Bible say that bodily exercise profits little?

First Timothy 4:8 is an interesting verse. We've talked about it before, but I want to highlight it here in a special way. They had bodily exercise every day. You'll recall that in Bible days people lived a life that was more intense physically than any gym today.

Jesus was a carpenter. He was a physical worker. They usually walked where they went. They had no power tools or electronic conveniences to do the heavy work. Life itself was a workout.

So when this Scripture verse was read by its original recipients, they would have recognized immediately that it was meant to be a comparison between the physical and the spiritual.

The physical is temporary; the spiritual is long lasting. Growing Christians know that their spiritual exercise is of more eternal value than even their physical exercise. Because while physical exercise benefits our temporary well-being on earth, spiritual exercise and spiritual health benefit our permanent, eternal well-being with God in heaven.

A TIME TO COMMIT YOURSELF

As we conclude this book, please read this passage from 2 Corinthians 7:1: "Therefore, having these promises, beloved, let us cleanse ourselves from all filthiness of the flesh and spirit, perfecting holiness in the fear of God." We have the tools now, the keys to our *Bod4God* lifestyle. So it's time for commitment. It's time to cleanse our bodies from all those things that would keep us from having a *Bod4God*. It's time for us to act on what we know to be true.

On page 117 is a commitment form. I want to challenge you today to make a commitment to having a *Bod4God*. I urge you to sign this commitment form and commit yourself to having a *Bod4God* lifestyle.

I've done my best to share God's Word with you. Now will you make a commitment to do it?

James 1:22 says, "But be doers of the word, and not hearers only, deceiving yourselves."

THE

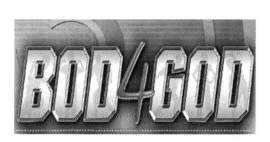

PLAN FOR YOU

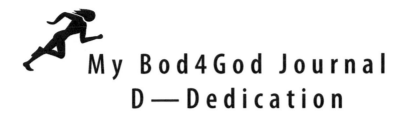

My Bod4God Journal
D—Dedication

I say then: Walk in the Spirit, and you shall not fulfill
the lust of the flesh.
(Gal. 5:16)

WHAT GOD TOLD ME ABOUT DEDICATION

_____

_____

_____

_____

_____

_____

_____

_____

_____

_____

_____

_____

_____

_____

_____

_____

_____

_____

_____

WHAT I'M GOING TO DO WITH WHAT I'VE LEARNED

_____

_____

_____

_____

_____

_____

_____

_____

_____

_____

_____

_____

_____

_____

_____

_____

_____

_____

_____

_____

_____

_____

_____

_____

_____

_____

_____

_____

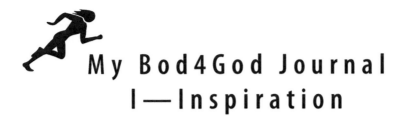

My Bod4God Journal
I—Inspiration

*The thief does not come except to steal, and to kill, and to destroy.
I have come that they may have life, and that they may have it
more abundantly.*
(John 10:10)

WHAT GOD TOLD ME ABOUT INSPIRATION

_____

_____

_____

_____

_____

_____

_____

_____

_____

_____

_____

_____

_____

_____

_____

_____

_____

_____

What I'm going to do with what I've Learned

_____

_____

_____

_____

_____

_____

_____

_____

_____

_____

_____

_____

_____

_____

_____

_____

_____

_____

_____

_____

_____

_____

_____

_____

_____

_____

_____

_____

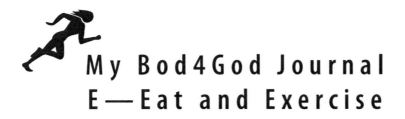

My Bod4God Journal
E—Eat and Exercise

That each of you should know how to possess his own vessel in sanctification and honor.
(1 Thess. 4:4)

WHAT GOD TOLD ME ABOUT EATING AND EXERCISING

_____

_____

_____

_____

_____

_____

_____

_____

_____

_____

_____

_____

_____

_____

_____

_____

_____

_____

_____

_____

WHAT I'M GOING TO DO WITH WHAT I'VE LEARNED

_____

_____

_____

_____

_____

_____

_____

_____

_____

_____

_____

_____

_____

_____

_____

_____

_____

_____

_____

_____

_____

_____

_____

_____

_____

_____

_____

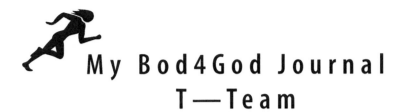

My Bod4God Journal
T—Team

*As iron sharpeneth iron, so a man sharpeneth the
countenance of his friend.*
(Prov. 27:17)

WHAT GOD TOLD ME ABOUT TEAMWORK

_____

_____

_____

_____

_____

_____

_____

_____

_____

_____

_____

_____

_____

_____

_____

_____

_____

_____

_____

_____

WHAT I'M GOING TO DO WITH WHAT I'VE LEARNED

My Bod4God Commitment Form

Dedication: Honoring God with My Body

I say then: Walk in the Spirit, and you shall not
fulfill the lust of the flesh.
(Gal. 5:16)

Inspiration: Motivating Myself for Change

The thief does not come except to steal, and to kill, and to destroy.
I have come that they may have life, and that they may have it
more abundantly.
(John 10:10)

Eat and Exercise: Managing My Habits

That each of you should know how to possess his own vessel in
sanctification and honor.
(1 Thess. 4:4)

Team: Building My Circle of Support

As iron sharpens iron, so a man sharpens the
countenance of his friend.
(Prov. 27:17)

KNOWING THAT MY BODY IS MADE BY GOD AND FOR GOD, I COMMIT MYSELF
TO A HEALTHY LIFESTYLE.

_____   _____
         Name   *Date*

*If you'd like more information about having Steve Reynolds
speak to your group, or conducting a Losing to Live Weight
Loss Competition, visit our website at:*

www.BOD4GOD.org

or write to:

*Bod4God
Capital Baptist Church
3504 Gallows Road
Annandale, Va. 22003*

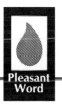

Printed in the United States
133302LV00003B/79-270/A